Moving Beyond the Unspoken Grief

A doctor's memoir of her own IVF journey as a patient

By Dr Sarah Lnyy

Dreamstone Publishing © 2016

www.dreamstonepublishing.com

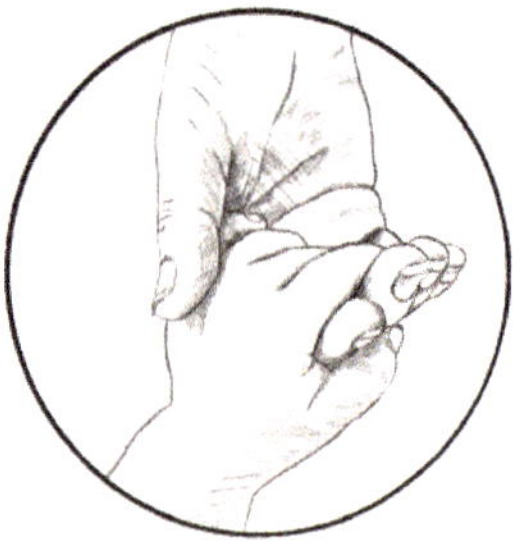

ISBN: 1925165949

ISBN-13: 978-1-925165-94-4

Disclaimer

The information, strategies, concepts, techniques and suggestions in this book are of a general nature only, and do not constitute, and are not intended as a substitute for, professional or individual advice in any way. You should consult with the appropriate qualified professionals (including psychologists, psychiatrists, counsellors, medical practitioners and other healthcare providers, insurance advisers, financial advisers, and legal advisers) and seek your own independent professional advice relating to your particular circumstances and needs.

Although the author and the publisher have made every effort to ensure that the contents of this book were accurate at press time, the author and the publisher do not represent or warrant their accuracy. The author and the publisher are not responsible for any disruption, loss or damage (including indirect or consequential damages) suffered by any party as a result of, or in relation to, the use of this book. To the extent permitted by law, the author and the publisher exclude any liability (including liability for negligence or other default) to any party for any disruption, loss or damage (including indirect or consequential damages) arising from or in relation to the use of this book.

What Readers Are Saying About This Book

"This is a candid and poignant memoir of how lives can be turned upside down in the journey to parenthood. Having a similar journey to Sarah, for no two IVF journeys are ever the same, I can relate to Sarah and Sam's rollercoaster ride. For some, it bears rich fruit, for others it can seem a never ending journey.

We were one of the lucky few to achieve our dreams of holding our child in our arms. As a medical practitioner, I had advised many on fertility issues but never thought I would end up needing help myself.

Sarah articulated the dichotomy between doctor and patient very well. Her writing is easy to read and engaging and had me cheering for her and Sam and I'm very glad to read of their bundle of joy."

– **Dr Bee Khuu, Specialist General Practitioner.**

"Infertility is an unexpected, punishing road of confusion, vulnerability and private turmoil. Sarah generously invites us into her turn on the rollercoaster. Honest and matter of fact, this diary, peppered with medical notes for the uninitiated, pierces the heart."

– Dr Tammy Brinsmead, Neonatologist.

"*Moving Beyond the Unspoken Grief* is a truthful and heartfelt account of a doctor's journey through the IVF process. Although armed with medical knowledge and experience as a doctor, Dr Sarah shows that perhaps there are some things in life for which one cannot be fully prepared."

– Ms Agatha Yim, Little Polly Pictures.

"I decided to read "Moving beyond the unspoken grief" because, while I'm surrounded by friends and clients who are travelling through the IVF journey, I know very little about it. This book made me laugh and cry along with Sarah and her quest for a family. This informative, rollercoaster of emotions helps tell the story of IVF and helped me to understand how hard it is for couples trying to conceive. Thank you so much for sharing your story with us, Sarah."

- Ms Lauren Brown, Founder of Lollaby, #nannyboss.

Table of Contents

Dedication

To my three IVF forum buddies on 'What to Expect', thank you for being there from day one. Although we have never met, through our correspondences, we shared one common goal and dream. It is hard for others to truly understand our journeys of ups and downs and this is one of the reasons I wrote this book. Congratulations on your successes. I look forward to meeting all of you and your expanding families.

To my acupuncture doctor, Dr Alice Gao, thank you for your tremendous support. Thank you for your guidance through traditional Chinese medicine and acupuncture. No one wants to be a pincushion, so thank you for being gentle with those long needles.

To all the staff at Epworth Richmond, Melbourne and Monash IVF, Dr Lynn Burmeister and my IVF nurses, Charlotte and Corrine. Thank you for your ongoing support during such difficult and emotional times.

To my dog, Andy, you always showered me with love and loyalty, making those failed attempts a little bit more bearable. Now, without you by my side, I know you will look after us from in Heaven above.

To my sister, Agy, thank you for being such an awesome sister. Your humour, comics, music and laughter brightened many dark and horrible days. There will be plenty more catch-ups over coffees and cakes.

To my parents, Herbert and Stella, thank you for giving me life and hope; for those endless trips going in and out of hospitals; for the constant supply of homemade soups on many rainy days – my heartfelt thank you.

To my darling husband, thank you for your support and endless praises of encouragement. I do not know how you have put up with the hormones. Thank you for your never-ending faith and commitment to our marriage.

*Note: The author has chosen *Dr Sarah Lnyy* as a pen name. Names have been changed in order to protect the privacy of the families and patients of the author.

Foreword

It is hard to be a woman in the modern world.

We are told that we can have it all. We can study, take on any profession we choose, build a career, marry, have a family, and keep building that career. The juggle is delicate and sometimes the balance is hard to find.

We tend to marry later more often than not, and actively choose to delay starting a family, until we are well established in both our careers and our marriages. More and more, professional women, who have listened to society's expectations and started down this path, struggle when it comes to having a baby.

Moving Beyond the Unspoken Grief achieves what most literature in this space fails to provide: both a heartfelt account of the IVF journey, and a clinical approach to describing the treatment processes and outcomes.

Dr Lnyy draws on her professional skills as a GP, trained in shared care obstetrics, to skillfully bring to light the reality of undergoing fertility treatment from a medical perspective while engaging the reader with her spiritual and emotional journey through the process.

While Dr Lnyy and her husband were fortunate enough to achieve their dreams of starting their own family, this book still provides a powerful reassurance and empathy for all women who experience fertility issues.

It takes women like Dr Lnyy, speaking out in this public way, to help normalise the reality of IVF in our everyday lives.

Maybe it's affecting the woman at the desk next to you; maybe it's affecting your best friend, but she's too heartbroken to open up to anyone about it. This book gives society a valuable insight into the importance of understanding the emotional rollercoaster that fertility treatments can create, and allows us to develop greater tolerance and empathy for our fellow sisters as they engage on their quest for motherhood.

Mary Sheargold,

Senior Associate at Prolegis Lawyers,

The Mac. Rob Foundation Limited

Prologue

Dear baby Babe,

I don't know whether I will ever hold you in my arms. I don't know if you will ever be born. If desperation and love and longing and perseverance could create you and implant you into my body, and keep you there, I would already have you nestled within me. For now, all I can do is write to you as if through the writing I will draw you to me.

To those embarking on this same path, who read this book - I do not know you. I have not had the opportunity to meet you. From the bottom of my heart, I wish you all the very best. I hope that you will find the most dedicated specialist team, having the best number of high quality embryos, the best outcome and the least affected with the unpleasant side effects. There will be many hopefuls and there will be many sorrows. There will be many wasted tears, wasted time and wasted embryos. The investment may never be returned as a bundle of joy.

Despite this, we choose to continue, cycle after cycle, in the hope of winning that pregnancy jackpot. In the end, there is an answer for us all. Seeking fertility treatments is a maze full of crossroads, corners and roadblocks. It is very easy to lose the sense of reality when you start to ponder about previous difficulties and failures. However, you do have the choice of letting go of the past. You can choose to live the present and look forward to tomorrow.

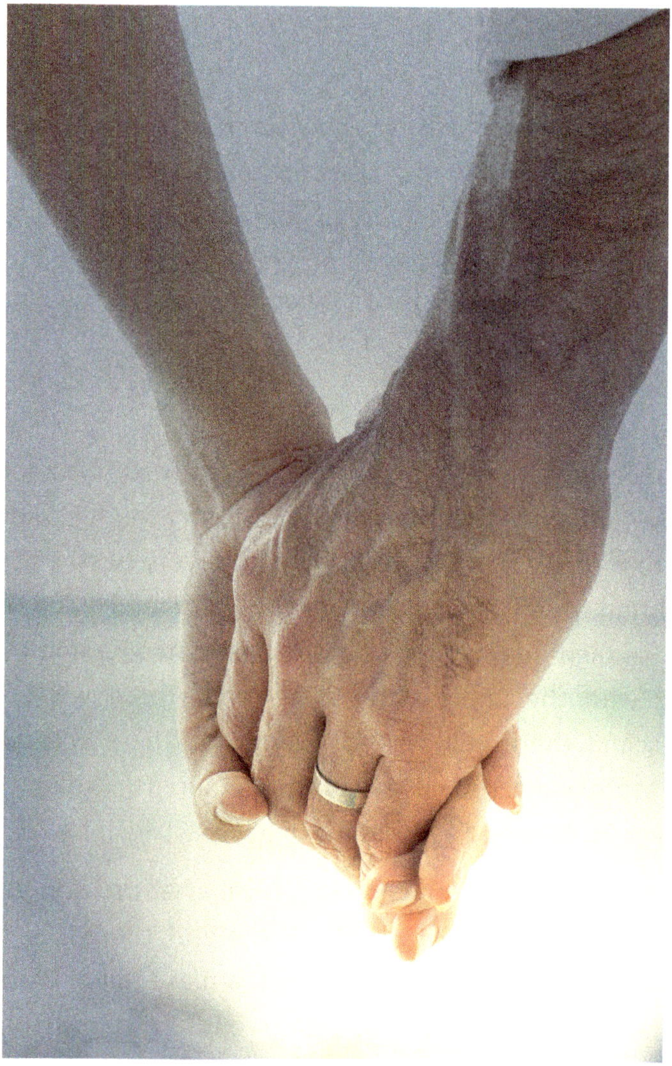

Chapter 1: First There Were Two...

From: Sarah

Subject: Are you there?

Date: 26 August 2011 10:37:52 PM AEST

To: baby Babe

Dear baby Babe,

Hope this email finds you well. I have recorded some personal videos a few months ago but decided that it is better to send you emails. Seeing me, your mum, on the screen may be a little bit confronting. Besides, people look a couple of kilos heavier on screen than in real life, right?

One day, I hope you will understand how special you are. I know you will have a zillion questions, so, these emails will give you an insight as to what was going on in our lives.

Today is 26th August 2011 and it is the day that I have set up this email account for you. I don't know if you will ever exist but we refuse to give up. When the time is right, I will hand over the email login and password to you.

Love, Sarah

This is how you began: An ordinary day. A normal stairwell. But, somewhere between the first and second floors on those concrete stairs in the Sunderland theatre building at Melbourne University, my life changed forever.

It was an afternoon between one long, second year medicine lecture and the next, and the stairwell was full of students from higher floors going down and from lower floors going up. A commingling of driven people either chatting noisily or with heads down, intent on getting to where they are going.

I noticed a guy about to pass me on his way down. He was good looking and had something about him that attracted my attention so, in a move quite out of character, I smiled and said 'Hi'. He seemed surprised, but smiled and said, Hi, how're you?' That was it – the tiny gesture on an otherwise unremarkable day in 1998 that started the whole wonderful, devastating, painful, glorious story of you.

A few days later I saw him in the library, and this time he made the first move by noticing that I was studying Biochemistry and recommending an excellent textbook on the subject. Because he was a year ahead of me, his advice was founded on recent experience. In the second week, Sam – by now I knew his name – asked me out to lunch. This was awkward because I'd agreed to go into the city with friends to see a movie. My hesitation was brief though, and I quickly ditched my friends for the sake of getting to know this guy better.

Over lunch we enjoyed that exciting 'first date information-sharing' thing, that can be the start of something deeper, or can just as easily sound the signal to run.

He discovered that I had been born in Hong Kong and arrived in Australia in 1989; I discovered that he had been born in Malaysia in the same year as me. It was clear from our lovely, long lunch that not only did we share similar values, so did our families. We talked about our parents, siblings, his childhood in Glen Iris and mine in Donvale; our life experiences (as much as we had gathered in our 19 years) and by the time we stepped back onto Royal Parade to return to the Faculty of Medicine, we both knew that we were going to see much more of each other.

And we did, baby. Any chance we got, but because we were both committed to our studies, our relationship was often conducted via phone calls, snatched between studying, lectures and exams. That was okay though. We understood each other's time allocations and focus completely, so when sightings were scarce, and face-to-face dates were scanty, neither of us felt sidelined. Our shared goal of graduating as doctors made things much easier. For four years we just kind of hung out.

The first three years of a medical degree is spent at university and the second three in clinical schools attached to hospitals. Sam was first to leave the walls of academia and begin his hospital General Medicine and Surgery year at The Austin Hospital in Heidelberg. By the time I arrived there, for the same rotation, he was ready to leave for his fifth year medical training rotations, at various hospitals across Melbourne and country Victoria.

And so it went – our clinical work sometimes throwing us together, sometimes flinging us apart. By the time Sam began his final year of internship, his attraction to work in anaesthetics was crystallising into something that would eventually become his passion.

Critical Care and ICU rotations paved the way, and when he applied for a position as anaesthetic registrar at the Austin – only a handful would be chosen from all of the hopefuls – he got it. I was so excited and proud. You've got such a clever dad.

In the meantime, I had been through the same rotations, but was forming the sense that general practice was singing to my soul. The Austin hospital residency rotation took me through Urology, Geriatrics, then Paediatrics at The Royal Children's Hospital then on to Northern Hospital for a Diploma of Obstetrics and Gynaecology. Of course, at that point I didn't know how the things I learned during that Diploma would one day consume my every waking moment. But that was still some years off – although I knew the facts of fertility and pregnancy, I was still an innocent in matters of personal experience.

It was 2006 before we could marry, confident in the knowledge that we had given everything we had to our studies and could now give everything we could to each other. Oh little one, it was the most gorgeous day. We booked the date a year in advance, unaware that it was the most propitious date for romance on the Chinese calendar.

Traditionally, many Chinese families will follow the Chinese Lunar calendar when it comes to celebrating important dates such as birthdays and picking the best date for wedding. Neither of us came from a very traditional Chinese family, so we had no idea that it was a kind of double Valentine's Day and only comes around every few years. Looking back, we realise that we were very lucky to be able to book a venue, because many Chinese couples had scrambled to get that date.

We were offered a cancellation. And so, with our careers set up and the Chinese calendar's enthusiastic approval, I walked down the aisle of the glorious Xavier College chapel, confident that our lives were blessed.

And in so many ways they were. In terms of weather, the day was the pick of that week. Whereas the days before and after our wedding day were around 15 degrees, our day was a sunny 26 degrees. This was fortunate because I wore a dress with spaghetti straps that would have been a very poor choice any other day that week. With family – many having travelled from overseas – and friends gathered around us, life seemed perfect. Photos from that day will show you just how happy we were, your Dad and I, bathed in warmth and sunshine of every sort.

We had bought a house in East Malvern, a year before, and had rented it out, but now we moved in and settled happily into married life. It was a given that we would start a family one day – Sam had already declared that he would like two children and that sounded good to me – but there was no hurry.

Sam was yet to sit for his fellowship exams and I was enjoying my GP work. I had never been terribly clucky, although I had enjoyed cuddling the little babies during my obstetrics rotation. We were young and fit. There would be time. We would simply call for you when we were ready and you would come to us.

After a couple of years spent this way, our thoughts turned to you, and in 2007, we began to plan for pregnancy. We were excited, imagining our lives as a trio. Although the first few months went by without sign of you, we were not worried.

Sometimes this happens after years of taking the pill, as I had done, since painful periods began it in my mid-twenties. In the first months that we didn't fall pregnant naturally, I just assumed that I had got the dates wrong or that we were physically stressed. Generally, if a couple is healthy and under 30, I would advise them to try up to 12 months. If they are in their early 30s they should try up to six months before undergoing investigations; from 35 onwards, about three months if there are no significant or relevant past medical history, otherwise the couple should be referred to specialists immediately. I was still under 30, so time was on my side.

Besides, Sam was diligently studying for his fellowship and working frequent night shifts. With me on days, our body clocks were as out of sync as our rosters. At the beginning of 2008 I made a New Year's resolution to get back to the gym and get fit and lose some weight in preparation for falling pregnant.

In January, I also started a skin cancer course, because I had begun to feel drawn to skin diseases as an area of practice. By February I had added a massage course. I found this to be a wonderful adjunct to my conventional GP skills because, while advising patients on pain relief, I was also able to provide hands-on targeted therapy for them. I honestly believe that this was the best therapy I ever offered in my General Practice.

This one had the double advantage of an additional skill to my repertoire (I was trying to learn as much as I could before starting a family) and a tool to help Sam de-stress during the run up to his Fellowship exams. He was treated to nightly massages which, of course, he loved. Such activities are very good for any relationship and we were starting to need it.

With our work schedules and Sam's study, the stress was telling on us both.

However, on 29 May 2008, he received word that he had passed and we were both over the moon. Back to serious planning for our baby.

While we waited for you, I took an introduction to cosmetic medicine and set my feet on a career path as a cosmetic physician. This is about art, symmetry and individual need. I learned that it was not about changing peoples' looks, but the enhancement and balancing of their best features and assets. I was one to encourage people to retain a natural look, rather than focusing on one specific area. I took to it happily because it is all about helping people with their confidence and self-esteem.

However, time was speeding by, and we began to wonder. The window of opportunity narrows as we age and tiny, barely perceptible doubts began to appear.

And of course, as time passed, other people began to wonder and ask. Their questions came easily, but answers were harder to find. Inquiries turned into sympathies for my childless state. Instantly, everyone became an expert in baby making. From sitting on a chair recently used by a pregnant woman to going on more holidays; from eating lots of Papaya to putting a newborn singlet under our mattress; from praying out loud every day to burning soya candles and almost setting the house on fire. There is nothing we didn't try. The priest who married us must have forgotten to pass on the bible of baby making.

I should have recalled the pain of my menstrual cycles and that should have been a warning sign.

This pain is so often a sign of endometriosis. Although I had never been diagnosed with this, had I thought about it, I might have started trying earlier. Oddly, we didn't think about that. We were doctors; we understood fertility; we just didn't necessarily apply that knowledge to our own situation. We were confident that you were waiting for us, just beyond the next month or two. But two years passed and you did not come. It was time to admit to ourselves, and each other, that something was wrong and that we had to seek help. It was time to euthanize any pride or ego. We made an appointment to see a gynaecologist.

Chapter 2: Life as a Doctor Wanting More

From: Sarah

Subject: It's a little hard

Date: 29 August 2011 09:25:32 PM AEST

To: baby Babe

Dear baby Babe,

I desperately wanted to cry at work today, but I stopped myself from doing so. I have been looking after a young pregnant patient, only to find out that she miscarried at an early stage. Her eyes were filled with sadness and I could only sympathize with her. I don't know if I would ever be pregnant. For now, I can only hope for the best.

Love, Sarah

I'd advised patients about fertility, pregnancy and all things baby-related, but now it was us. In general practice, I specialized in student health, women's health and pregnancy care. I have shared tears with patients and witnessed many joys and sorrows. I can relate to many couples undergoing assisted reproductive treatments. Sadly, about one third of them ended up in separation and later, bitter divorce. It is a constant reminder that we are only human, and our existence is fragile.

It was January 2010 before I could see my gynaecologist, who was thorough and professional. She ordered many tests and during the next few months I had blood tests, each of which returned an NAD – No Abnormalities Detected – result. We were advised to make some lifestyle modifications to improve our chances of success. We did everything asked of us. Still nothing happened. I tried not to self-diagnose or self-treat. Being doctors did not spare Sam and me from the harsh reality of infertility and the tricky and often gruelling work of assisted reproduction.

Although we are equipped with medical knowledge, contrary to a common misconception, it does not make the process easier. I could not fall pregnant faster than other people. I could not distance myself from the sadness; I could not use my medical knowledge to soften the blows of losing the chance of you, month after month.

In fact, in many ways, being a doctor made things worse for me. My practice, at a university student health centre, was varied and interesting. Patients were a mix of people, with the usual medical complaints, and I saw all the harder to fix problems, such as homesickness, loneliness, relationship issues and a myriad of other problems that beset students.

Students often felt lost in the huge institution, were juggling part-time jobs and classes while all the while trying to enjoy the post-school freedom that they had longed for, throughout their teens. A great number of them were living away from home for the first time – many dealing with living in the city, while missing their families in the country.

Not that they would present with 'homesickness' or 'broken off with partner' or 'panic over exams' at the beginning of our doctor/patient relationship, but I could usually see when constant headaches, lethargy, panic attacks or similar were symptoms of some larger problem. I wanted to know what was happening for them in their broader lives and so I would gently probe. Gradually their stories would emerge. Many in the student cohort of any large, city university need a compassionate ear as much as they do a stethoscope.

However, because of the nature and age of the patients, a recurring presentation was unwanted pregnancy. It became harder and harder for me to deal with this. Some wanted themselves relieved of the 'burden' others chose to see the pregnancy through. It was not for me to judge the rightness or wrongness of their decision, but wanting a child as much as I did, these cases broke my heart.

Take Mary (not her real name), she was a high school student, accompanied by her boyfriend who was two years her senior. Within five minutes, a simple urine test convinced all of us that she was pregnant.

The idea of being a young father proved too much for the boyfriend and dealing with an unplanned pregnancy seemed too much for Mary without his support.

Sadly, as a result, they split up a few days later and, worst of all, she was kicked out and left homeless by her boyfriend's family, who wanted nothing to do with her and the unborn child.

A week after the blood tests, Mary returned alone for follow up. According to her blood work, she was about six weeks pregnant. The stress, solitude and fear had taken their toll on Mary – she'd aged almost ten years since I last saw her, a week earlier, and had definitely lost a few kilos. I was extremely concerned for her welfare.

She confided in me that she was using alcohol and smoking as her way of relieving stress. My heart sank as I sent an electronic internal memo to my receptionist, informing her that I would be running late with my schedule. After much discussion, Mary bravely decided to continue with the pregnancy.

"This is it," she said. "This is my calling. Now, I have the responsibility to look after something of my own." She said it with a forced smile but determined eyes. It was her decision, and her right, to choose to continue with the pregnancy. Mary promised to cut down on smoking, stop drinking alcohol and cease any further drug use. I referred her for an early pregnancy dating ultrasound to pinpoint her exact gestation and, most importantly, to check the wellbeing of the foetus.

I still remembered the day when I downloaded her ultrasound report from the computer. There was a dull ache in my heart and I felt sick in my stomach. Sadly, the foetus stopped growing around the time of the six-week gestation. Mary had not had any bleeding but there was no foetal heartbeat. It was a contained miscarriage. Upon revealing the results to her, she cried with such devastation. We both grieved for the loss of her tiny angel.

While providing as much emotional support as I could, I felt my own heart breaking. I wanted you so badly and my tears were for her loss, but also your continued absence.

Genetic abnormality seemed to be the commonest cause for miscarriages in early pregnancy. However, I also discussed other possible contributing factors such as extreme stress, drug use and fluctuations in hormonal imbalance. I referred her to The Women's Hospital for a follow up procedure. A few weeks later she returned for a review. She looked older than her age and underweight. She wished to have some closure and wanted to find out the hospital policy on handling the remains of the miscarriage. To be honest, I had no idea. Nobody has ever asked this question and when I worked as a resident in the hospital, I had never thought about this.

After several phone calls, I spoke to a lovely lady from The Women's Hospital. Whilst admitting it was rather an unusual request of information, she understood our concerns and informed me that all the lost Angels are cremated. The ashes are scattered in a special area located in the Lilydale cemetery. She gave me instructions on how to locate the sacred area. I passed on the details to Mary and she thanked me as her eyes were filled with tears. Mary was the bravest young woman I have ever met. Within the outer fragile shell, there was a strong determined young woman. This has brought closure for both of us and I was humbled by this whole experience. Mary was an inspiration.

Sam and I needed that kind of strength, and sometimes strength is in accepting defeat and asking for help. It was that time for me, so I went to see a colleague whom I had worked with when I was a resident in the hospital.

I confided in her and she took me under her wing. There were many tests, both for me and for your father, various pathology tests and intrusive questions. Although these things were difficult, they finally revealed the answer: there were, indeed, issues that meant we would not conceive on our own. It was not the answer we wanted, but it was an answer that could paradoxically move us forward, hopefully closer to you.

We were referred to Melbourne IVF and I had my first appointment on 23 June 2011.

Chapter 3: Unexplained

From: Sarah

Subject: I dreamt about you

Date: 30th August 2011 04:25:34 PM AEST

To: baby Babe

Dear baby Babe,

I had a dream about you last night. We were in a park and you were chasing the birds with our dog, Andy. I watched you from a distance and you two were having so much fun! In my dream, you wore a pink ribbon in your hair. You were dancing and spinning around in a floral red dress. You ran towards me, holding out your hands and wanting a cuddle. In my dream, you were a little girl.

Do dreams come true?

Love, Sarah

All our tests were repeated after six months of modifying our lifestyle, in order to improve our chances of success.

It was a cool day, but not cold, when I made my way into the Melbourne IVF clinic specialist's rooms. I always attended the consultations on my own, not because Sam did not want to be there, but because, as an anaesthetist, he was needed elsewhere. His anaesthetic lists were demanding, and as a doctor's spouse, I had come to an early realisation that his days were mostly given up to his patients, and I'd already accepted this as part of life.

As much as it would have been nice for him to accompany me, I was quite comfortable attending on my own. As for Sam, he trusted me and knew that, with my medical background, I would understand the medical jargon and the plan of action to follow.

So, I was on my own when I found out that I couldn't conceive naturally. 'Unexplained'. That was the answer the specialist gave me to my question of why. Our initial tests had been normal, but apparently a small percentage of patients (approximately three per cent at that time) were diagnosed with "Unexplained" infertility. It was more difficult for younger couples to accept when the cause cannot be explained. For the older couples, age and the quality of the eggs made the issue a little clearer, and their situation perhaps more predictable.

Unexplained was not an explanation of any sort – it felt unsatisfactory. To this day, I think she meant to say, "We have yet to find the cause, so keep trying". Back in the good old medical school days, one of my predecessors once told me "things are often missed, not because of not knowing, but rather because of not looking hard enough".

Keeping this in mind, we had held onto this never-ending ribbon of hope, with absolutely no guarantee. Now we had to begin again, sailing into an unknown phase of our journey, hoping that it was guiding us towards parenthood and you.

I left the specialist's room feeling confused, frustrated, angry and guilty. Confused at the diagnosis of 'Unexplained'.

Surely there had to be an explanation to everything. I was frustrated because I dealt in facts and 'unexplained' was not a fact – it was a very poor adjective. I was angry that we had to deal with this, when baby making shouldn't have to be like that, and I felt distressed because, deep down inside, I felt "NQR" - Not Quite Right. I knew that no one could treat an unexplained condition. With no explanation, we had no clear way forward.

These feelings were soon joined by others. I felt sad, and somewhat guilty: perhaps we should have tried even earlier. I was angry because we had chosen a profession where, in the beginning, with our careers still in limbo during the long years of our training, we had delayed thoughts of parenthood. I thought of all those years of being on the pill for painful menses – had that done more harm than good? Obviously, I was experiencing the sort of self-doubt and recrimination that many women in my situation go through, because I knew pretty well that these thoughts were purely emotional and not backed up by scientific evidence.

When I went home and discussed the diagnosis with Sam, he was shocked. Like me, he could not comprehend the diagnosis of 'unexplained'. He also knew that one could not treat an unknown cause.

At least, if it was something identifiable, we could target and work on it, and get to the bottom of things. We held each other, really overwhelmed and frustrated that our own fertility was beyond our control and that our fate was probably going to be determined by the trial and error of in vitro fertilisation - IVF.

I had left the specialist's rooms with instructions and a wad of papers. She instructed me to talk to Sam about IVF – our (apparently only) option. Should this interest us, then we should go through the papers she'd given me – information on IVF. If we decided to go ahead, we were told to complete all the paper work then organise a police check; a working with children check; make an appointment with a counsellor, another with a nurse, and another with the accounts manager, all in preparation for our first cycle of IVF.

Where I live, in the state of Victoria, Australia, you must have a National Police Record and Child Protection checks before being accepted into the fertility clinic program. Yes, pristine background checks. The certificate confirming that I was, indeed, a law-abiding citizen landed joyfully in the letterbox a week after my application. Weeks went by though, with no sign of your father's triple "A" citizenship rating. Was he really who he claimed to be?

If I hadn't known him for so long, I would have hired a private detective to do a background check on him. Six weeks later, the long-awaited certificate arrived and Sam sighed with relief. What a coincidence that someone with the same first and last name, living in a completely different state, had an extensive criminal record!

Chapter 4: Setting Forth

From: Sarah

Subject: Day 3

Date: 3rd September 2011 12:05:33 PM AEST

To: baby Babe

Dear baby Babe,

I started the injections today! It was a little bit harder than I expected. I prepared and laid out everything on the kitchen bench top. However, I found myself holding the injection pen and staring at the long needle for a few minutes. It must have been my imagination because the needle looked way too big for its job.

Luckily, your Aunty Agy was on Video Skype from London, so I was able to do the jab with her support and encouragement. We ended up talking for over an hour. Aunty Agy now calls me Jabba the Hut, hopefully not because of how I would look like. I have to jab myself daily for the next eight days. Fingers crossed that I will be ok by the end of these injections! Now, four hours down the track, I am already feeling quite bloated.

Hoping for lots of eggs for collection.

Love, Sarah

Our first two IVF cycles are called the antagonist cycles. I met with the nurse who oversees the process and made notes about what to do and what to expect. She needed to know about my body and I needed to understand the world into which I was about to plunge Sam and myself.

Her explanation went like this:

On the first day of my next period, I must call her to activate the IVF antagonist cycle.

On Day 3 I will start the daily injection of Follicle Stimulating Hormone (FSH) –a hormone that boosts the size and number of the eggs in the ovaries.

On Day 8 I must have an internal pelvic ultrasound to check the eggs' sizes and if there are not enough, or they are not big enough, I will continue with an increasing dose. If over stimulated, there is a chance that I will have to stop, to prevent a condition known as Ovarian Hyperstimulating Sydrome (OHS) which, at its most severe, can be fatal. It has sent some women to the intensive care unit for intubation, so the ultrasound is vital.

Two days before the Egg Collection procedure, I will have another scan to ensure that the follicles (the sacs that cocoon the eggs) are big enough and the numbers are good. If everything is as it should be, I will continue with daily FSH injection, plus the Antagonist injection (to prevent the sudden release of the eggs from the follicles), while I wait for them to mature.

Exactly 36 hours before the egg collection, I must stop the antagonist and FSH injections, replacing them with an HCG injection, known as the Trigger injection. This will release the eggs within the 36 hrs, in time for the egg collection.

On Egg Collection Day I will undergo surgical removal of the eggs under general anaesthesia. The eggs will be fertilised with the sperms.

Three days after that, I will go back in for the all-important transfer of the newly created embryo from the laboratory to me. Once the transfer has been made, I will have to apply progesterone vaginal cream for 14 days until the day of the blood test, regardless of whether I have any bleeding or not.

It was a lot to absorb, and I wondered how women with no medical knowledge find it.

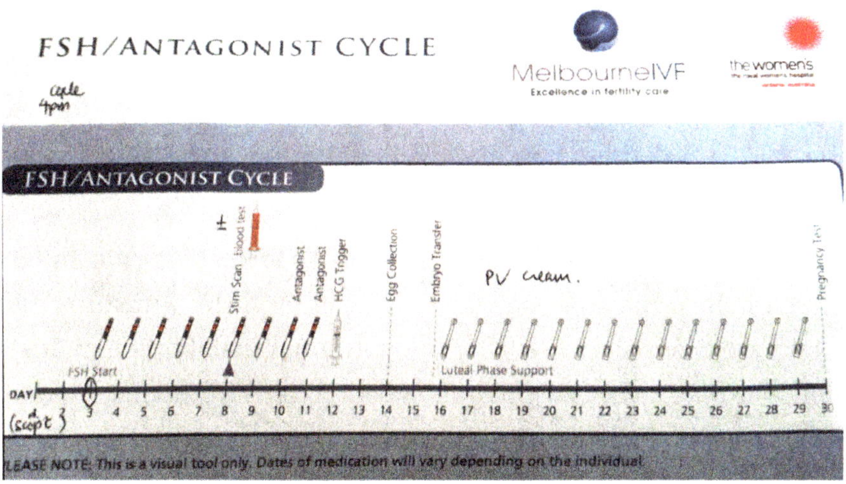

A time-line of the Antagonist cycle back in 2011.
This is a visual tool only and may have been changed since 2011.

Cycle one start date: 1 September 2011. This was the first day of my menstrual cycle and time to begin the complicated process. I dialled the nurse's number and she quickly summarised what I needed to do during the next two weeks.

She has no doubt given these instructions hundreds of times to hundreds of other would-be mums. Despite the meeting and notes, despite reading all of the information I was given – and more – at that point it was still just that, information. With this call, it morphed into my life. I listened intently to all she said and then I was on my own.

And so I began: on Day Three I sat on my bed with the first injection hovering over my abdomen, then plunged it into my tummy. It was painful – not the self-administered prick of the needle – but the medication inside.

The trick is to ice the injection site beforehand and to rotate the injection area on my tummy. It hurt a little less, but it still wasn't pleasant. I knew that this was the first of many, because I had to inject myself daily until the eggs were ready for harvest. During the trials, the fertility injections helped to boost my ovaries – my mini egg factories.

The timing had to be precise, even if I had to hide and inject myself behind the steering wheel in a car park. This reminded me of my medical student days, visiting a drug rehabilitation centre. Only this time, I was the patient, injecting furtively, hoping no one would notice.

By the end of the injection week, my tummy looked as if I had been in a motor vehicle accident. I had hit a small blood vessel and it bled so much that the bruised area covered the lower belly from the belly button down. Purple, brown, yellow and orange pigment artistically scattered all over the surface of the abdomen – my own abdominal Impressionist masterpiece.

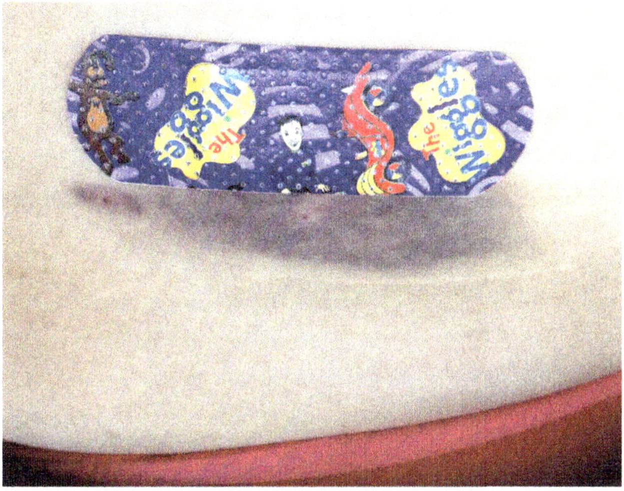

I was short on bandaids, and ended up raiding the kids supply at the clinic!

The first scan went well, then came the one that would identify the size and number of follicles that were right for harvest.

Each follicle, visualised on the scan, will normally house an invisible egg. The follicle enlarges as the egg matures within. They want to see a high number of large follicles, hence better chances of collecting good quality eggs.

Yet it's a juggling act between quantity and quality. Sometimes there is a dilemma: if there is only one large mature follicle, should you harvest that and have just one chance, or should you give it up and wait for the other eggs to grow, so that you have quantity on your side? The chance of success increases with a higher number of good quality eggs and this second scan reveals which of the stimulated follicles are producing. It is always a numbers' game. I had two.

14 September, 2011: Egg Collection day. Two things must happen on Collection Day: the precious specimen donated by your father must be delivered on time and in perfect order, and I must have my eggs harvested ready for their date with Sam's sperm, and our destiny. On the day of the egg collection, the husband would normally accompany the wife to the day surgery.

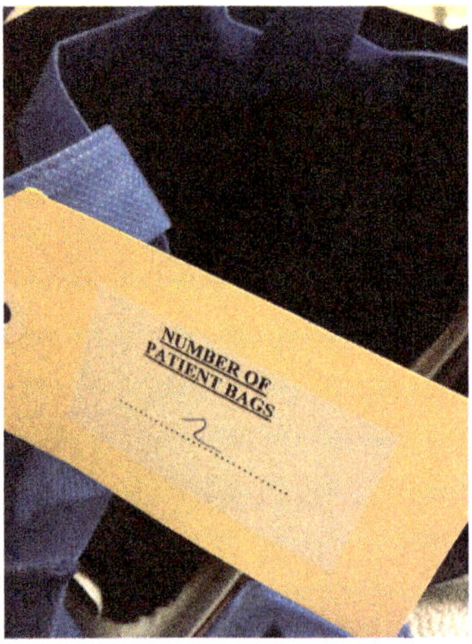

Pre op 'baggage'

The wife will be in the holding bay getting ready for theatre while the husband is guided to the "donation" room. Once the husband has a fresh specimen he hands it to the embryology team who will wash and prepare the sperm for insemination straight after the egg collection.

As it was impossible for Sam to take a day off from his theatre anaesthetic list, I brought his donation in with me.

The embryology team had told me that I would have one hour to deliver the specimen (in a jar, placed in a sock and cradled in my pocket) before the sperm denatures (loses its natural and essential qualities). So, I was very tense and rushed on the day of the egg collection.

Then it was my turn. I felt like a fairy-tale goose – as if the sole purpose of my life was to produce tiny golden eggs.

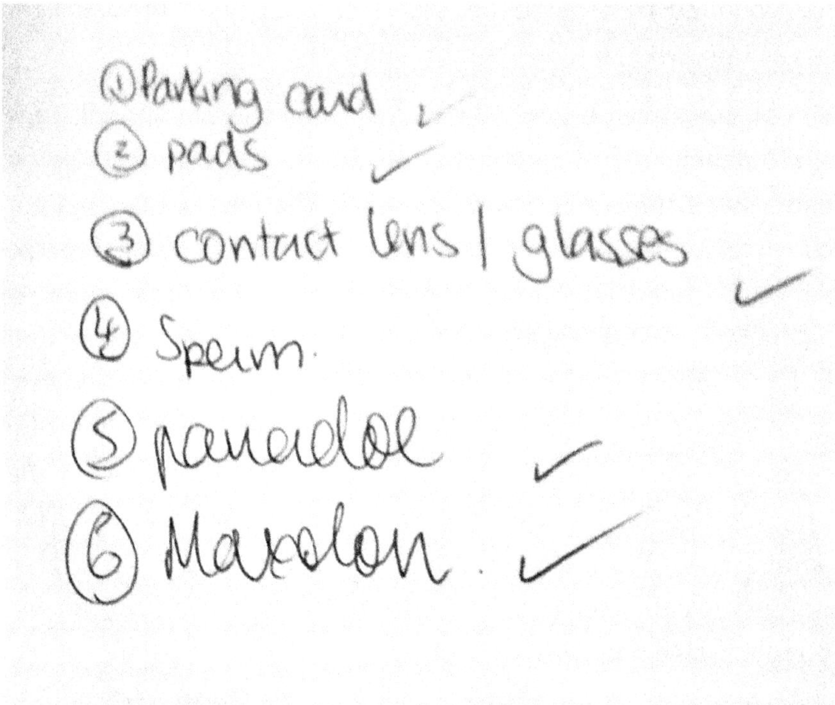

'To Do' List on the day of egg collection

Performance was everything. I was absolutely present, yet oddly detached:

Curtains are drawn and a spotlight lands on a woman in centre stage. She appears to be carrying a precious cargo in a tiny yellow capped specimen jar, stored in a pair of warm old woollen socks. After a quick exchange of words, she hands the container to the lab technician. As she makes an exit, she glances over a row of men queuing up to deliver 'their goods'. Some of them blushed and avoided eye contact. The air is still and the silence is embarrassingly uncomfortable.

The theatre is bright, spacious and cold. She shivers inside the thin patient gown as the spotlight lands on her white robes. Soon, she is surrounded by a parade of actors and actresses in their light blue scrubs, white kitchen hats and hippy booties.

With all eyes fixed on her, she makes small shuffling bridal steps on the imaginary red carpet, tiptoeing onto the theatre table on centre stage. With one hand, she holds the front of the patient gown and with the other, the ties on her back, being ever so cautious to avoid accidentally "mooning" the other performers. As she hops onto the table, the well-rehearsed and orchestrated staff attend to her every need. Blood pressure cuff on one arm, digital monitor on one finger. The oxygen mask reminds her of a scene with Darth Vader - *'You underestimate the power of the dark side'.* With that thought, the anaesthetist (with invisible vampire teeth) carefully examines her arm in search of a large juicy vein. Within seconds, she enters the dark side, lost in time and space, sleeping without dreams.

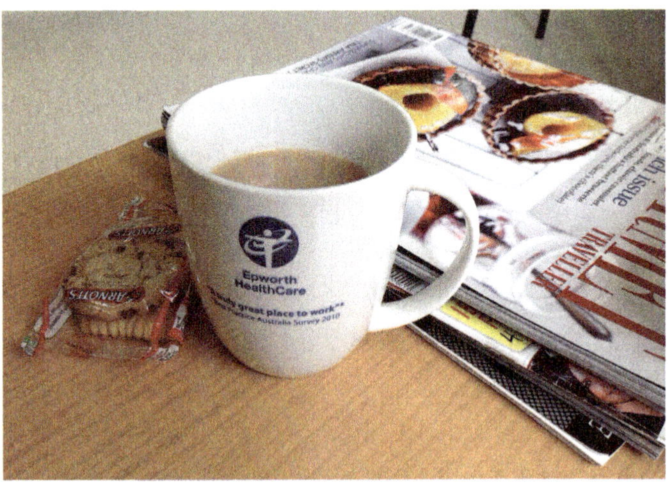

Post op recovery cuppa.

I woke up knowing that our sperm and egg were nearby in the midst of their whirlwind romance.

The marriage of egg and sperm complete, the embryologists baby-sat my fertilized embryos for the next few days, before recommending the best performer for the fresh transfer. To avoid a twin pregnancy, we have chosen to have just one transferred and have the rest frozen for later use.

Transfer day: 16 September, 2011, the day that the embryo was transferred into my uterus. This is when a precious embryo cargo makes its way back into the mothership womb where the magic really begins. I had prepared by going through the ritual of detox and sprinkling myself with sticky baby dust. On that day I returned to the hospital, only this time, I was ushered to the day treatment room.

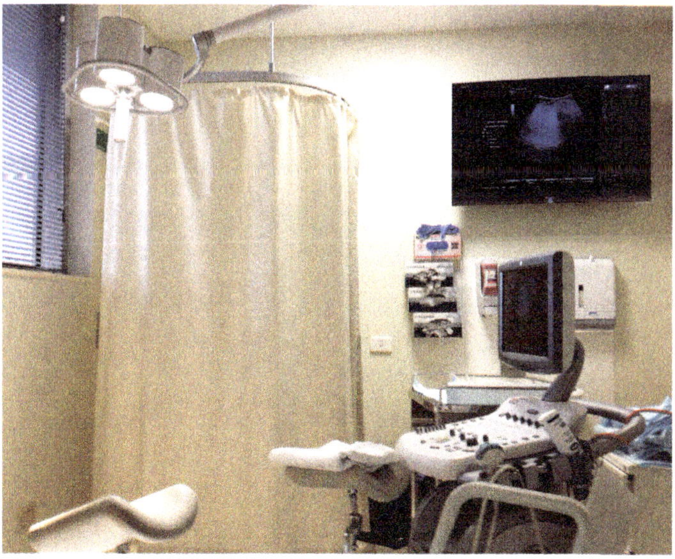

Embryo Transfer Procedure Room

Two important things must happen at the time of transfer: a full bladder (so they could visualise the area of implantation under ultrasound) and keeping very still.

This part was done without anaesthetics. With my legs wide apart, a twenty minutes procedure seemed like a lifetime. I closed my eyes, twiddled my thumbs, trying to meditate and relax.

Lying on the surgical bed perfectly still, I had dreams of you, in the same arena of hope. The embryos were ready but they only transferred one and kept the others frozen for the next round, should this one fail.

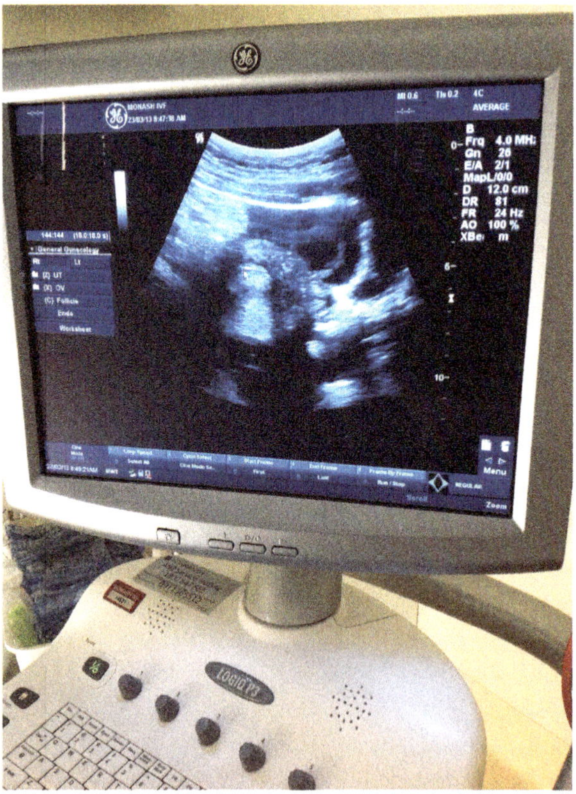

Different views in the Embryo Transfer Room

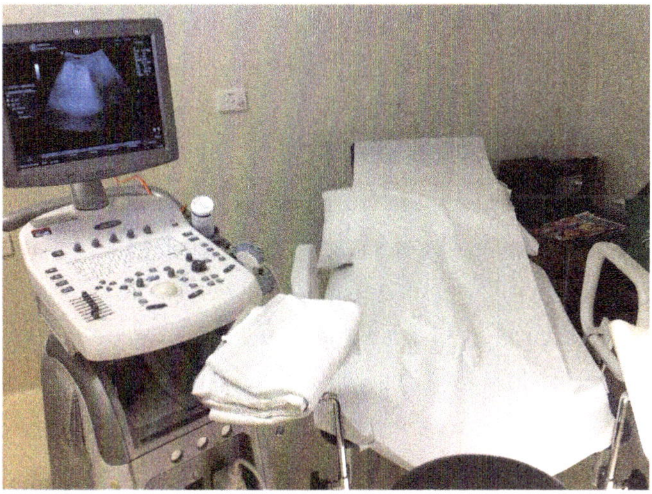

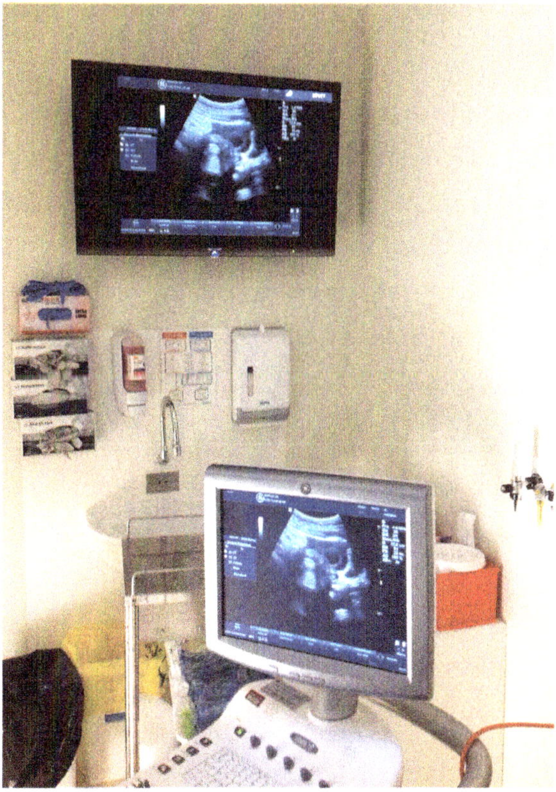

When I opened my eyes, I knew that, for the first time, I carried a tiny life inside me. Transfer is just that – the transfer of embryo from laboratory to uterus – it does not guarantee that the embryo will implant itself into the uterine wall. It would be two weeks before we knew whether it would attach and grow into you. So we waited to see if our best efforts and love had translated into a life capable of living outside a glass dish. For Sam and me, that very first two-week wait was the hardest. Our days were roller coasters of emotions. Paralysing. Sometimes it was hard to breathe. No matter how many times the doctors and nurses told me to *'carry on with your life as normal'*, I knew that I would never feel normal again.

My mind kept asking itself, *'Am I pregnant?'* My heart wanted it to happen so badly that my judgment and insights were often eclipsed by my blinding need. My medical knowledge became complicit in my fantasy. I looked for, and found, symptoms that convinced me that I was exhibiting early signs of pregnancy, but deep inside I knew that these were probably phantom symptoms, brought on by the side effects of the medications, and an overactive imagination.

It is best to avoid the Internet. I knew that, but I was as guilty as any layperson that wanted answers. I spent every waking moment in search of forums and blogs on topics related to what I was experiencing throughout the day. Before I knew it, seconds and minutes, then hours disappeared. Days were lost in the wonder of that ultimate question, *'Am I pregnant?'* but the answer remained elusive.

In the world of medicine and general practice, we can only help those who are willing to help themselves.

The same can be applied here, because genuine help is abundant if only you will ask.

Instead, I asked Dr Google. I also had another source of virtual support.

'What to Expect' is one the largest online public forums, for parents-to-be, worldwide. It is a place where anxious insomniacs, like myself, gather to discuss and vent about anything related to fertility, pregnancy and childbirth. In 2010 I had become a regular visitor. The idea of being anonymous and starting a conversation with a stranger did not bother me. In fact, it was a safe haven and an emotional outlet. I figured that, if I came across any eccentric people, I could simply log off and disappear. In fact, not knowing each other made it easier for everyone – a vehicle to catharsis and access to unseen supportive shoulders.

I started a new thread in the forum and only a handful of people responded to the discussion.

In the end, there were only four of us who would post regularly. We came from different walks of life, unaware of how our lives would be thrown into chaos. Sadly, each of us was an affirming statistic of the one in six affected by infertility. We had no knowledge of each other's existence until fate brought us together, yet here we were, bonding and sharing. After a few months, we decided it was time to partially reveal our identity and swapped email addresses. I soon discovered that we all reside in various States within Australia. What are the odds?

My first needle...' was the title of the thread where we first had shared our stories. We were all undergoing the first round of fertility drug treatments.

Comparing notes and treatment protocols, I remembered telling the ladies how much I hated giving myself the injections. Numbing cream would be handy, but I would use up an entire tube within a few days.

These women were so brave, as none of them flinched at the sight of the needles. Being a doctor myself, I should have been better at this.

Did you know that you could lessen the pain by icing the area for thirty seconds prior to the injection? The following is my two-cent's worth of advice to the others in the little group.

- Respect the needle. Don't be playful and start jabbing with the other hand.
- Respect the protocol. Don't start giving yourself more than required.
- Respect the "Me time". Don't rush. Find a nice quiet area for some time-out.
- Respect the body. Don't keep poking at the same area.
- Respect and involve your partner, only if he or she is not faint-hearted. Ensure that your partner is paying attention and not watching television. Make sure he or she warns you first with these three little words, *one, two, three*; followed by, I love you.
- Respect the moment. Don't laugh when the needle is in, it hurts more.
- Aim at an angle. Following the direction of the bevel can reduce bruising.
- If all else fails, grab the chubbiest bit of flesh around the waist, take a deep breath, go for it, and remember, breathe!

We had all endured our fair share of the emotional roller coaster, although this was certainly no amusement park. We were willing to risk it all – our physical health, our mental wellbeing, our jobs, our lives and potentially our relationships with our partners.

These were testing times.

United by one mutual goal and sharing one common dream, the four of us corresponded regularly, via emails, in emotional rain, hail or shine. I took comfort in sharing my journey with these ladies. They were pillars of strength despite my only having known them for a brief period of time. Weeks, months and years passed, four became three. Three became two. Two became one. Finally, I was left behind on my own. The only one not pregnant. Complete failure.

The feeling was worse than failing an exam despite studying diligently.

To this day, I still have flashbacks to more than fifteen years ago, the day of the fifth year Psychiatry exam. Within the time limit of an hour, I was instructed to take a detailed history from a patient and to present the case findings, with differential diagnoses, to the examiners.

Despite having an interest in psychiatry and having studied fairly consistently throughout the term, nothing would ever prepare me for the day. Nothing, except a spare battery, a pair of shoes and an adult diaper – these would have been handy.

I spent the first thirty minutes wondering why I could not communicate with the patient. Catatonic Parkinsonism? This was certainly not a case for a fifth year medical student.

It was only when I started scribbling on a large piece of paper, hoping that he could see through his thick broken spectacles, he eventually told me that he could not hear because his hearing aid died that very morning.

Oh for a battery. He could not see, as he was legally blind.

The last thirty minutes was spent trying to locate his shoes, so that I could help him make it, at a slow shuffling gait, to the bathroom. He had wet his pants by accident in the midst of laughing at my silent monologue interrogation. How embarrassing.

While making his way to the bathroom, he claimed to have more helpers up his sleeves, as he was the ex-Prime Minister of Australia. Keating? Hawke? Fraser? Whitlam?

Who else could it be? I flipped open his drug chart, glanced at the list of medications, located the patient label on the top right corner, and that did not help. I could not recall if there was indeed an ex-Prime Minister of Australia with the surname, *Smith*.

Delusional grandiose with Parkinsonism or Bipolar disorder. I stated these diagnoses during the case discussion.

Unfortunately, I did not mention any of these diagnoses in the case presentation. I overheard the conversation and a disappointing decision as I was closing the door behind the examiners,

"Are you seriously going to fail her?"

"Of course! She didn't include anyone of these as the differential diagnoses."

"But she presented the case under such difficult circumstances."

"That's just the way it is."

Trying in vain to remember the names of previous Prime Ministers, I regretted not taking political science as a major in medical school. I could not believe I was to list former Prime Ministers in a Psychiatry exam.

The patient possessed neither the first nor surname of any ex-Prime Ministers of Australia that I knew of.

The thought of failing this exam was very real. After wiping an entire body volume of tears off my face, I finally found some courage and started typing, and sent a fax to the faculty of psychiatry, explaining the appalling circumstances of the exam and details of the conversation between the examiners. Feeling deflated and exhausted, I buried my head in the books and tried to get some light reading in, before the written exam on the following morning.

Daylight came and I dragged my aching body out of bed. My goodness, how could one age so quickly overnight? Trying to put the frustration and disappointment behind me, I knew I had to refocus and concentrate in the written exam, even if it was only worth thirty per cent of the total mark. Surprisingly, once I put the pen on the paper, I found myself sitting in a fish bowl and my mind was impenetrable – nothing existed except the words I was writing.

At the sound of the bell, pens down! It was all over. As I was leaving the examination hall, a white envelope was waved at me from a distance.

With a letter of encouragement, and a few kind words from my supervisor, the Head of Psychiatry Unit, I did not expect to receive a faculty pass for my efforts in the case presentation. But, indeed, that was what the envelope contained.

It turned out if the examiners are to fail a student, they have to present and explain their reasons to the rest of the teaching panel. My letter had arrived just in time before the hearing. The lucky stars were on my side. I am prepared to admit that I was not the brightest amongst my medical peers.

I was not the cream of the crop, but I was hard working. Medical training has taught me a few things.

How often are we prepared for the unprepared? How soon do we expect the unexpected? Life is about meeting expectations and developing resilience when these are not met. I do hope that one day, I will join the ladies from the forum, expecting.

But I am jumping ahead of myself – let me get back to telling you about that first cycle.

Chapter 5: Prayers Answered

From: Sarah

Subject: Transfer completed

Date: 16 September 2011 9:06:52 PM AEST

To: God and baby Babe

Dear God and baby Babe,

Transfer completed. I am dusting myself with all the sticky vibes and pray that it will be successful. We won't know until two weeks' time. Meanwhile, I just have to sit tight with fingers, toes, eyes, legs... everything crossed.

I hope our prayers will be answered.

Love, Sarah

During this longest fortnight in history, my Dad was scheduled to have an elective surgery. His surgery was successful and unremarkable but, when he returned home, he became increasingly ill and I received a distressed phone call from my mother. I listened, with growing alarm, as she described the extreme pain and bleeding that had sent him to the emergency department, yet I tried to reassure her.

"Alright mum, I will go to the emergency department now. I will be there with you in forty-five minutes." I hung up the phone, rushed to my car and out into the peak hour traffic.

I found my father in one of the emergency cubicles. He had forgotten to withhold his blood thinners after the surgery and once he returned home, began to take all his usual medications. Now he was bleeding. He was stark white and his patient gown was bright red. The front was saturated with blood. And it didn't stop there – blood splattered across on the patient and cannulating trolleys, and pooled on the floor. Think horror movie.

I had a quick word with the attending emergency doctor and the urology registrar on duty that day. The plan was for my Dad to be transferred to a private hospital nearby, once he was stabilized. But for now it was a battle for stabilisation.

Severe cramps started in my lower abdomen.

While I worried about him, my father, as always, worried about me.

"I am so sorry. I hope I haven't worried you, especially as you have just had your transfer a few days ago." Dad spoke with such sorrowful and guilty eyes.

He was quite short of breath from the loss of blood and was in obvious pain.

More cramps.

I took slow deep breaths, trying to calm myself down. They were in vain. As I was speaking to the Urology registrar, Dad had a hypotensive episode and passed out in his chair. Instead of lying flat, resting his frail body on the bed in the emergency cubicle, dad had been led to a neighbouring chair by a nurse, so that the nursing staff could change the blood-soaked bed sheets.

No one expected Dad to collapse.

Luckily, Mum was with him at the time and triggered the emergency button. Within seconds, a dozen staff from the medical and nursing team rushed into the cubicle and worked on him.

There is a reason why doctors should never treat their family members. Witnessing my Dad's hypotensive episode was extremely stressful. My legs felt like jelly and I could feel myself trembling inside. I started to bargain and prayed: "Dear God, please look after my Dad and let him pull through. I would rather see my Dad live and recover fully, more than anything else." I prayed hard with tears streaming down my face.

And the cramps persisted.

My father's condition stabilized after a few units of blood transfusion. He then experienced an episode of angina from fluid overload and was given diuretics.

As for me, my prayers were answered.

My father survived, however, I bled later that night and for us, it was a Big Fat Negative (BFN).

My notes tell the story: Bled: 28/9/11. I'd had cramps a few days after transfer and they increased in frequency and intensity throughout the second week. The blood test had confirmed it: my worst fears: negative. It did not work. I was not pregnant.

I sobbed during most of my waking hours. I cried in hiding during the day. I wept as I fell asleep.

Andy, my dog-child, licked my tears away in the hope of offering some comfort and solace. This faithful and loyal Maltese X Silky could only survey the devastation of the battlefield. Perhaps, being a dog parent would be the closest thing I would ever be. I tried putting on a bright face each morning, only the tears would ruin the day's makeup.

Our world stopped and we stood alone inside a time suspension capsule. The outside world, unaware of the pain and suffering of its occupants, would keep on revolving, day after day. We pushed on, already planning our next journey into purgatory.

Little one, life itself is a miraculous gift. It can give you so much wonder, joy and pain. When it comes, welcome it with all your heart and soul, because life is so very fragile.

Chapter 6: Coping in General Practice

From: Sarah

Subject: Miracle pending?

Date: 30 September 2011 9:34:50 PM AEDT

To: baby Babe, God

Dear baby Babe and God,

As expected, no good news today.

I guess it's not the right time.

Sigh.

I am getting better at dealing with bad news though. I think your father is still pretty angry and upset. This is really hitting him hard. As I was driving on my way home today, a song was playing on the radio... '...what doesn't kill us will only make us stronger'.

You know, there is some truth to it.

We have been praying for a miracle. However, it seems there isn't going to be an early Christmas present for us now. We will try again next cycle.

Love, Sarah

"Excuse me. Why can't I get an appointment with her? I am pregnant and she is the only one in this clinic who can provide shared care. She cancelled last week too. This is ridiculous! She is so unreliable. I am going somewhere else!" One of my patients complained over the phone to the receptionist.

This was apparently the standard response of a few of my antenatal patients when told I wasn't available for an appointment. The IVF procedures and the days leading up to the transfer had been extremely stressful.

I was jamming my blood tests and scans into cracks in my working schedule and often spent too long in other people's waiting rooms. This meant getting back to work late for appointments.

Then there would be times where an extra blood test and further ultrasounds had to be scheduled at specific times of the week. I had no choice but to reluctantly cancel many general practice sessions at the last minute.

It was obvious that every day in general practice was a constant battle. The sudden cancellation of the general practice sessions was nothing but disruptive for the practice and for my patients. I have always been an organized person, and I could not bear letting these patients down. This was certainly disruptive, distressing and unforgivable.

Fortunately, my practice manager and the receptionists were very understanding. I had informed them of what we were going through and they were very respectful and supportive.

I wished some of my patients would understand that doctors are not super heroes or heroines.

We were not immune to illnesses, failures and disappointments.

A young married couple came in after a miscarriage at 18 weeks gestation for advice. Sadly, the miscarriage was found to be due to a rare chromosomal abnormality of the foetus.

Unfortunately, this was not diagnosed through the earlier routine blood work. Constantly reminding them that it was not due to something that they had or had not done, I could sense their guilt and self-blame. I referred then to a fertility specialist for ongoing management.

A few months later, I was surprised to see the wife, this time on her own, requesting a form of contraception prescription. The couple had divorced soon after having their first cycle of fertility treatment.

A lot of things surfaced while they were undergoing treatment and they realized that they were no longer compatible.

The treatments were also disruptive to their lives and difficult, both physically and emotionally.

It dawned on me that our own fertility journey was not just about me. Although it was my body at the centre of our hopes, our dreams of parenthood and our disappointments were equal.

It made me realise that I might have neglected Sam's mental wellbeing all of this time.

The last time I wrote a love letter to my husband was when we were dating as medical students.

It was time for another:

Dear Honey,

Words cannot explain what we have gone through in the last few months. Thank you for your constant support and taking part in this special journey with me. At times, I feel scared and lonely because of the unknown, and, at other times, due to the intense pain as the direct result of all the procedures and medications. There are times I am so frustrated that I just want to lie in bed all day, burying my head and have a good cry. This whole experience has been so emotionally overwhelming that I am gasping for air.

I have been emotionally labile from the unfriendly hormones; the side effects are so unpredictable. I feel our lives are spinning more and more out of control. Socializing less and trying to avoid places with children are my only two options. I know this is silly, but this is my way of self-preservation. Whilst dealing with all the internal pain and the hostility of the outside world, the hardest part for both of us is dealing with other people's comments about our childless state.

To this date, I hate the fact that I am always the one breaking the bad news to you. I will never forget the disappointed and deflated look in your eyes. Over and over again, I have let you down.

I know you are hurting too, despite this, you continue to encourage me and remind me that everything will be all right as long as we have each other. Without love, we will never succeed in this human love project.

I am beginning to understand that the World will keep on revolving with or without us. Tomorrow is the future that has yet to be written. I know there are no guarantees to any successful IVF story. With a glimmer of hope and a burner full of love, I know we can count on each other in continuing this crazy journey. Ultimately, when the time is right, we will finally accept and surrender to our fate.

Lots of love,

Your little pincushion.

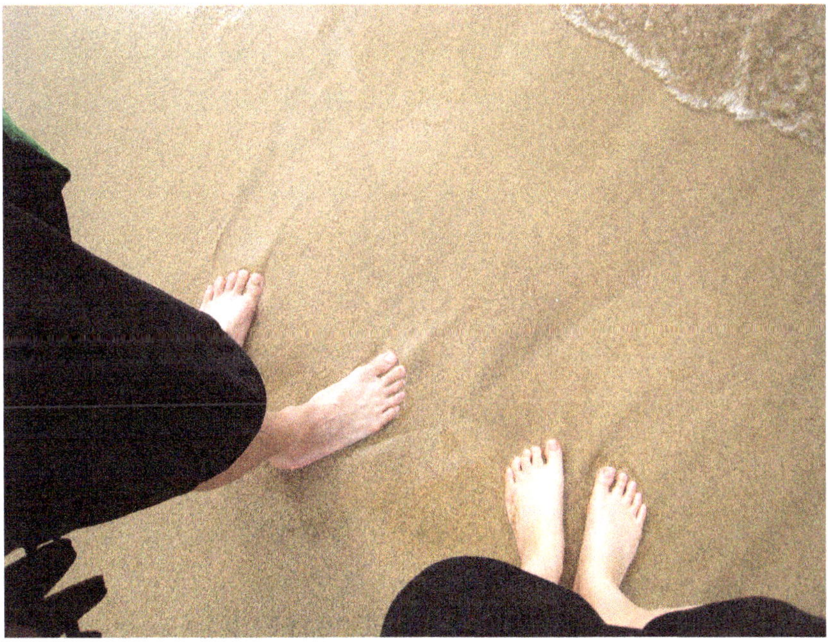

Walking together.

After reading my letter, your dad broke down and so did I.

We discussed our fears and planned for our future. This whole experience had brought us closer.

He has always been my rock. No matter how sad, crazy, unpredictable or anxious I was, during this mad scramble for you, he was my Guardian Angel. He will make you the most wonderful dad.

Chapter 7: Continuing Our Battle

From: Sarah

Subject: Embryo Transfer today

Date: 17 November 2011 12:20:11 PM AEDT

To: baby Babe, God

Dear baby Babe and God,

The egg collection occurred three days ago. The embryo transfer happened this morning. We made it! Your dad could finally come with me to see exactly what happens at the transfer. It was a wonderful experience for him to finally get the chance to view the embryo on the screen.

We are not greedy, just one will do.

Blood test will be scheduled on Friday in two weeks. Fingers crossed.

Thank you, God, for looking after me throughout this journey. I pray for all other couples who are going through the same process and hopefully they, too, will soon have some good news.

Love, Sarah

All that we were going through might be considered a self-inflicted torture. Mostly, I felt that it was a battlefield.

The first battle had been lost, so we gathered what little strength we had left, psyched ourselves up, and got ready for the next strategic plan of attack and the next battle. We never doubted that you would be worth it.

Meanwhile, the other two embryos from the first cycle waited, frozen in time.

The second attempt began two months after the first, and just six weeks after our first failed embryo transfer (it is not considered a miscarriage as the embryo has not implanted. Any failed implantation is not considered a pregnancy).

The first day of my menstrual cycle, 4 November 2011, began with the instructions to use a different medication in the place of FSH (Follicle Stimulating Hormone).

This time I would take Clomiphene, which, like FSH, is an ovarian stimulant but it is less intense – which was fine because we did not need to harvest eggs.

Otherwise, it seemed like a re-run of the first cycle: good scans, but only two promising embryos this time.

Sam and I decided that we would increase our chances of success by transferring both embryos and, so, I walked into the day procedure treatment room on 17 November 2011.

Were we hopeful?

Yes, why not? We had doubled our chances and that had to be good.

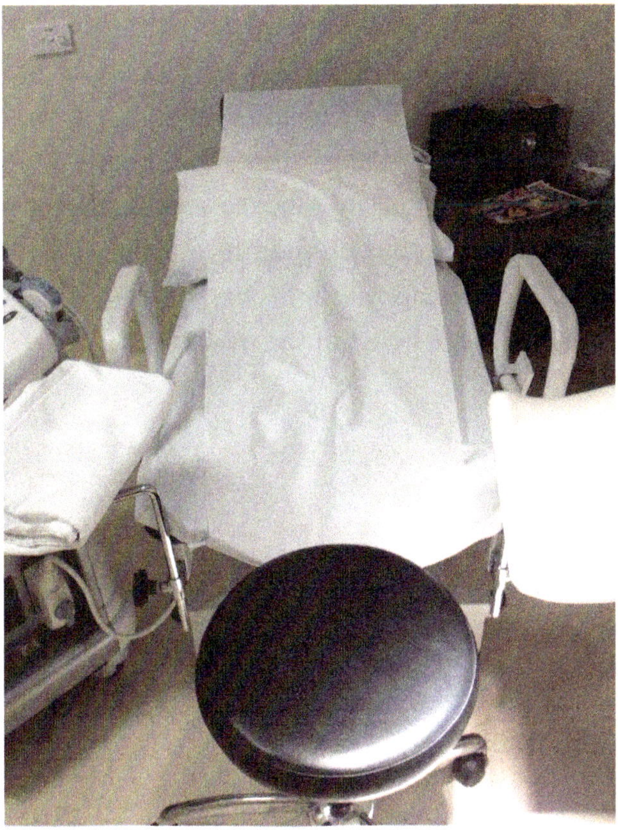

Getting ready for another embryo transfer

We waited again. A week passed and all looked good, despite some light cramping which could have been hormonal.

One week down, one to go.

During the second week of the two-weeks-wait, cramps were becoming more frequent and intense.

They were very similar to the cramps just before the arrival of my period, which I had always called Aunt Flo.

In order to distract myself, from what might or might not be happening inside my body, I decided to take up a hobby. This helped to clear and refresh my mind - I called it a 'brain enema'. I recovered the sewing machine that had been sitting in the cupboard for years. After doing some research online, I took an e-sewing lesson on the web. I decided to make cushions, lots and lots of them. The sewing machine was running day and night, sometimes into the wee hours of the morning.

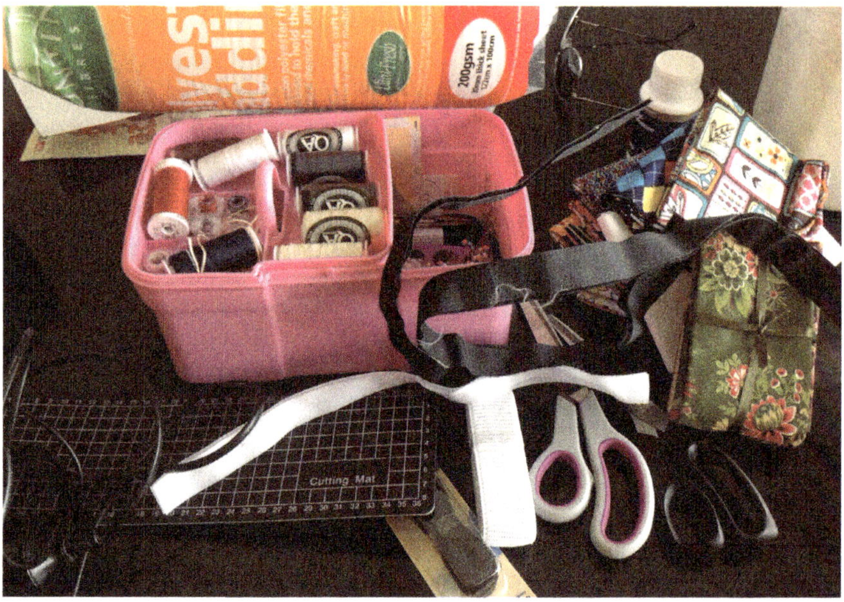

My Sewing Kit

We ended up with lots of new pillows and cushions all over the house and in my parents' home. Once the cushion craze ended, I took up photography. Through the lens of the beholder, it engaged me to look at life differently, to capture the essence of the day and be blown away by the beauty of Mother Nature.

During this time I was moving too fast, trying to outrun the waiting time. My thoughts were racing and the only way to quieten my inner fears and hopes was to fill every corner of my waking hours with activity.

Two weeks went by and the time was up. I had a blood test scheduled to take place on 3 December, 2011, to determine whether this had been a successful attempt. So much time, money and emotion had been invested in such a short period of time. My emotions were on overdrive when I arrived at the IVF pathology centre. There were many nervous women and their partners waiting for the pathology nurse.

Of course, I slept poorly the night before, partly due to the extra progesterone support and also from thinking too much. The other women looked no better than I did.

"Could this be the day?" I kept thinking over and over again. The good news was that Aunt Flo had not arrived. I was secretly hopeful.

The waiting area was very small and crowed. There were only a handful of chairs to be shared with other women waiting for their embryo transfers. I picked up a pathology number in the queue and sat down quietly in the corner of the room.

Suddenly, I had the most severe and excruciating cramp. I quickly rushed to the lavatory adjacent to the pathology room.

To my horror, I bled. I flooded. The entire toilet bowl was filled with bright red, angry blood. I had my period, which meant that almost certainly, neither embryo had implanted and I was not pregnant.

I was completely paralysed. Shocked, devastated, frightened, angry and guilty. Every emotion hit me at once as I began to sob, hunched over in the confines of the tiny toilet cubicle.

Realizing that only a few centimetres of plasterboard separated me and my anguish from the pathology room, I buried my face in my hands, trying to contain and suppress my grief and disappointment. I have never felt so alone. This was one of the lowest points in my life. This Aunt Flo was not kind; the cramps and bleeding continued for a long time.

Somehow, I found whatever strength and dignity I had left inside me. I tidied up, put on my sunnies and returned to the waiting room, to face the harsh and unforgiving reality.

The waiting room seemed a lot smaller. As I sat myself down again, a woman pushed her pram into the waiting area. She took a number from the queue - she was waiting for a blood test. Her child started to play with her toys and making loud giggling noises in the centre of the room. I wanted to get up and leave, to be anywhere but there.

I just wanted to hide somewhere to have a good cry. There were a few quick glances from the other women in the waiting room towards the child – some of resentment, more of yearning. It was quite a painful sight to bear, knowing for certain that this attempt had failed.

I was finally called for the blood test. The nurse would contact me on my phone within a few hours. *'Is it going to be a BFN (Big Fat Negative) or BFP (Big Fat Positive)? Please, let it be a BFP!'* I prayed very hard, although I already knew the answer. Tic, toc; tic, toc; tic, toc.

I counted every second that went by. My life revolved around the clock, the hormones, Aunt Flo and this moment. Finally my mobile rang.

"I am so sorry to inform you that the pregnancy test is negative. You are not pregnant. Have you got an appointment to see your specialist for a follow up?" Though it was no fault of the nurse, she apologized profusely. I fought back the tears and swallowed hard, falsely reassuring her that I was fine.

'Suck it up!' I said to myself. *'This must be some sort of punishment for whatever terrible things you have done in your past life.'* This horrible thought crossed my mind and I hated myself. My husband had gone to work particularly happy because it was blood test day – he, too was secretly hopeful that we would finally have some good news.

Now he was on the other side of town waiting for my call. I could not imagine how I was going to be able to make that single phone call that would destroy his dreams. I reached for the phone.

"It's okay sweetie. We will just try again." He spoke with so much sadness in his voice. When he returned home from work, he hugged me as I sobbed uncontrollably, for what felt like a lifetime. We grieved over the loss of our perfect embryos. There were so many unanswered questions.

First stimulated cycle: failed. First frozen embryo transfer: failed. Second frozen embryo transfer: failed.

Aunt Flo arrived mercilessness and punctually towards the end of each two-weeks-wait. It was a love and hate relationship with her.

When a transfer failed, I would hate to see her angry red proof of failure but I could also see her as the first day of the next cycle of hope. The hate gradually became stronger than the hope.

We returned to work, which helped both of us to refocus and regain some momentum in our lives. It took a while before we could discuss our lost hopes and plans for the future.

Chapter 8: Dealing with Other People

From: Sarah

Subject: Big Fat Negative BFN second cycle

Date: 29 December 2011 7:06:01 PM AEDT

To: baby Babe, Mighty God

Dear baby Babe and God,

We have had a lovely Christmas and I cooked dinner for about ten people. Aunty Agy came back from London, Cousin Ann visited from HK with her two friends, Aunty Mary and Pat were here to celebrate Christmas with us. Unfortunately, I bled heavily just before Christmas. It was negative again. This means I can probably finish off all the different types of cheese in the fridge right now.

The lucky stars weren't on my side this time but I do hope that someone else has won the pregnancy lotto. I have booked myself in for a review on the 9th of Jan and will see how we go. The nurse said my doctor would generally want to wait for a month after a stimulated cycle before commencing another cycle. However, at the transfer, my doctor told me that she could start me on the thaw cycle straight away.

I am not sure now. It has been pretty tough for me emotionally lately. If a marriage survives IVF, it can survive most things.

Love, Sarah

"Hello! This is 'Amy' from The Blood Bank. How are you today?"

"Yeah, good thanks." I lied. I found it easier to tell a white lie than to explain that I was actually feeling absolutely horrible. It had only been a day since finding out that our sixth attempt had not worked. My eyes were still puffy from crying. At least it got rid of some of the wrinkles around my eyes.

"This is just a courtesy call to let you know that our mobile blood bank will be located near you in the coming weeks. Would you like to make an appointment for blood donation now?" It was a very young voice over the phone and she spoke with such enthusiasm.

"I am sorry but I won't be able to donate now as I am currently on an IVF program. I have just had a zillion blood tests." I replied honestly and politely.

"Oh! (Long pause) I see, so how long have you been doing this program and when will you be able to donate again?" Amy asked innocently.

My blood boiled. I was flabbergasted at her naïve and insensitive questions. Remaining calm and collected, I replied that it was something private and I did not wish to discuss it with anyone.

"Hang on, I will put you through to the nurse right now." She replied. Without asking my consent to transfer the call, she directed it to a nurse. Feeling rather frustrated and angry, I complained to the nurse that it was nobody's business but mine, and they couldn't intrude like that into people's private lives. The nurse was very apologetic and understood that this had created unnecessary stress and distress.

She kindly took me off their calling list, at least for a couple of years. Perhaps it was a simple misunderstanding. Perhaps it was my raging hormones. Those three little letters - IVF – meant so little to some, yet so much more to others.

The truth was, that while our lives were in a desperate holding pattern, others' lives went on and while that was only right, sometimes it made things hard for us. I couldn't pretend that everything was fine when I sent RSVPs to children's birthday parties. Inevitably, you are caught off guard and have babies thrown onto your lap by unsuspecting new parents, followed by innocent but heart-piercing comments like, "oh look at you, you are so clucky" or "you will be a perfect mum, one day".

I learned to say "No thanks" for the sake of my mental wellbeing in that delicate time.

As for the people who were already standing on the lucky bridge, I am sorry. You probably thought that I had disappeared from the face of the Earth, or was just too busy with my own life, and couldn't be bothered. I don't blame you for not understanding. It is not something I shared openly, because every failure took a toll on my heart and soul. My heart was frozen and my horizon closed. This was my way of survival. In those days, I learned not to judge people, because we do not comprehend the struggles behind each human facade.

Then there were the marvellous moments and I found great comfort in my parents. They had migrated to Australia in 1989. They loved Australia and wanted to provide a better future and opportunity for their children. My father is a very conservative and traditional Chinese man.

He is a man of not many words, yet his pearls of wisdom sometimes surprise us all.

"In this day and age, there are many children without proper parental guidance and support. Some of these children grow up to become troubled adults. The world has changed and it has become more and more challenging to raise children. Your mum and I will always support you. No matter what happens, you can count on us to be there for you. We just want you to be happy and lead a healthy life. You don't have to have children and be a parent to lead a fulfilling life. We have always been proud of who you are and what you have become."

I drew strength and courage from these words of wisdom from my father. Little one, my wish is that someday I will be able to share my father's wisdom with you and my grandchildren.

I drew strength from this, but the longing would not recede, so counting the day in the pathology collection centre as the first day of my next menstrual cycle, I began the next IVF cycle almost immediately – 4 December 2011. A new round of injections and scans followed – a merry-go round with which I was becoming sadly familiar. My eggs were collected on 15 December, they were transferred two days later and again, just before Christmas, I discovered that this attempt too, had failed.

That Christmas, I went to evening Mass. It would be the last time I went inside the Church. Having suffered another failed treatment, I had doubts about whether God actually existed. As I sat down quietly with your father, I was approached by a local parishioner, requesting us to carry baby Jesus and present it at the Altar with the entrance of the procession.

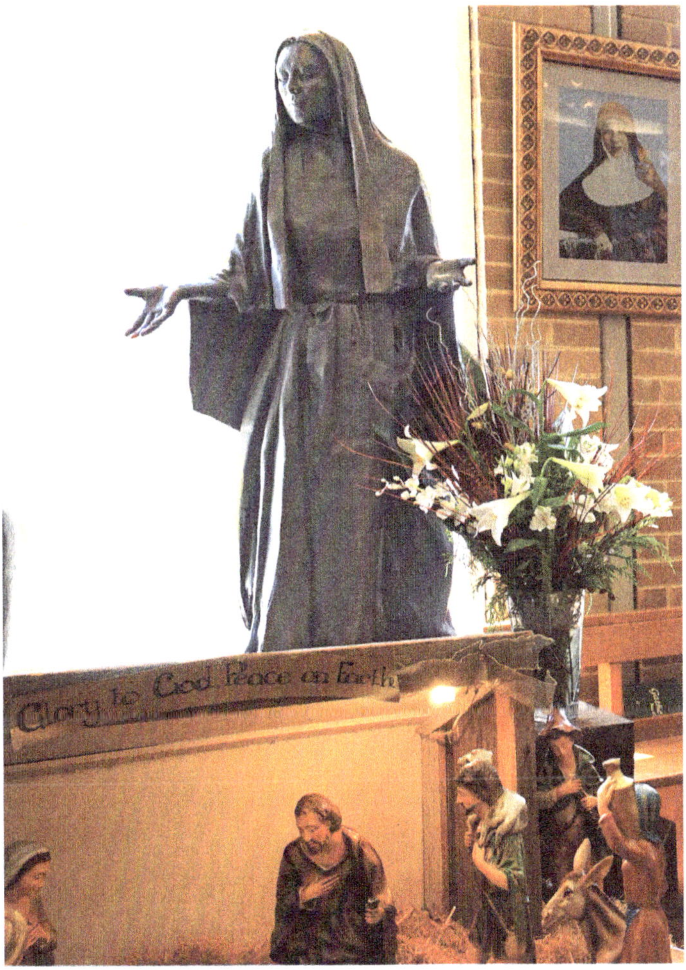

Why me?

It was worse than rubbing salt into the wound. I felt like my heart was stabbed a dozen times. I politely declined without giving a reason but she was very insistent.

Why, in a hall jammed packed with churchgoers, were we the chosen ones? I spared your dad from walking down the aisle. I was afraid that he would never attend mass with me again. As I looked down at my palms, holding baby Jesus, I felt the weight of my feet and the heaviness in my heart. How could life be so cruel? I was so upset. I vowed that I would not step one foot into the Church ever again. Was it a tease? Or was it a sign of comfort and solace? I couldn't say. I didn't know what to think but acted upon how I felt at the time.

Chapter 9: The Gap Year

From: Sarah

Subject: Happy Valentine's day

Date: 18 February 2012 11:36:35 PM AEDT

To: baby Babe

Dear baby Babe,

Two cycles have passed, six embryos have failed to implant and have gone to heaven. We are taking a gap year as a drug-free holiday!

It was Valentine's Day on Wednesday. I finished work early and went to get some flowers for my mum and mother-in-law. Luckily, I got home early, as your dad had secretly arranged ten red long-stem roses to be delivered at the door. He is so sweet. Oh so well trained!

Right now, as I am typing this email, your dad and I are lying on the floor of the alfresco watching the stars of the night. He has downloaded this app from the Apple Store that helps you to identify all of the stars in the sky. When you are old enough, mummy and daddy will show you the World and its beauty. It's truly magnificent! Life is beautiful.

Love, Sarah

"Daddy, can you tie my hair up.... please?"

"Turn around darling. Sit down. Look at how soft your hair is! It smells so good! Did mummy use something nice for your hair?"

The child giggled as her dad, like a pro, tied her hair up in a ponytail in the blink of an eye. Impressive.

I observed the reaction of my husband. His eyes were filled with sadness, and a dash of envy.

He decided: "Right now, the only thing missing is my life is having a child of my own. In twenty years' time, I don't want to look back and regret, if only we had tried harder."

Looking at Andy waddling at a stately, geriatric pace along the park, I had nodded.

"I had never thought having kids would be so difficult. The last two cycles have really traumatized me. I wouldn't start another cycle right now; I may be ready in a couple of months. You know, this IVF thing, there is no guarantee. When do you stop? I am really scared that there is no end point. You lose control of everything."

"When will we be ever ready to try again to be parents?" He had pulled Andy aside from the footpath to give way to the little girl riding a tricycle. There were four pairs of eyes full of admiration.

In recent news, a test has been developed to offer better success in IVF treatments. This complicated test involved checking the genetic material of an embryo before it is transferred back into the woman. If an abnormality was found, the affected embryo would not be used for the transfer.

In order to proceed with this selection, the couple must undergo further compulsory counselling sessions where the psychologist discusses the procedure.

Furthermore, they have to make an advance decision on the outcome of the embryos, in the event that one or both parties suddenly pass away. We have not really thought of our own mortality apart from the time when we visited our solicitor's office, setting up our wills and power of attorneys for each other. We would be more than happy for the other to use the remaining embryos with our respective future partners, should either one of us have kicked the bucket first.

Out of pocket expenses would be about $3400. In addition, we must also sign a consent form, agreeing that we will not engage in any sexual activity, to eliminate the possibility of a natural conception occurring without prior embryo genetic testing. This was to protect the IVF provider, in case the couple conceived naturally with a child affected by genetic abnormalities.

Confusing? If this entire journey has been overwhelming, this has certainly raised the bar to another level. To procreate, we must abstain?

We deferred the testing - apart from the distress and confusion, I had long felt burdened as the bearer of both the embryo and the ultimate, disappointing, news. One might think that I would get used to giving the news of failure to my husband. On the contrary, it was unimaginably painful every time. I felt so guilty because I was always the person who made that call. After going through many boxes of Kleenex, it took a lot of guts, tremendous inner strength and profound courage to be able to deliver bad news, over and over again.

Yet paradoxically, I also felt numb, as if the cumulative effects of the anaesthetic drugs had paralysed my true emotions. The more I tried to contain my disappointment and fears, the more withdrawn I became. As the treatments continued, I subconsciously trained myself to suppress a lot of anger, frustration and disappointment. My outer and stronger self would overshadow my inner and fragile soul.

Of course, there were positives and negatives to having acquired this newfound skill. The positive was having developed a defence, a self-preservation mechanism, in order to survive the ongoing failures. Unfortunately, it was affecting our marriage. My stoic suppression of emotions and feelings, in order to avoid conflicts and unutterably sad setbacks, kept people at arms' length – even my loving partner. It was truly a recipe to marital disaster.

I did not realize what was happening, until your father brought this to my attention. We finally talked. We argued. We grieved. Our guilt, regrets, and fears surfaced. I cried and we embraced the harsh reality and the unknown future. This was when and where the mending of our relationship began. I understood the need to be patient, to answer his questions, to alleviate his fears and listen to his worries. It was vital that I not brush aside these important elements. Sometimes I had already explored these issues myself, but it was vital for him to go through the same process of grieving and healing.

Although we might not have had all of the answers, we knew that we must listen to one another, grieve together and explore other options. No matter how hard and painful this journey had become, we knew we had to make time for one another, always following our hearts and keeping in tune with our feelings.

Battered and bruised, both of us had stumbled through this journey. Fortunately, one of us always recognized the danger and was able to alert the other. Much credit to Sam, he dusted me off and bandaged my wounds. It was a very valuable lesson to learn as a couple. One should not deny each other's opportunity to express his or her feeling. It was the route to taking charge of your life and to becoming a better person in a better partnership.

Our IVF journey was all about ups and downs, falling and getting back on our feet. If one of us was leading, getting too far ahead of the other, it was imperative to be patient and wait. We could not risk the danger that we would start to walk in the opposite direction. By then, it might be too late. We could end up saying to one another, "this is just too hard".

So after two years, two unsuccessful cycles and transfers, we decided to take a break from it all. I was desperately in need of a holiday from the invasive tests and the side effects of the medications. Recurrent IVF was hard on my body – the raging hormones and the repeated anaesthetics take their toll. Emotionally, the toll is possibly higher, if a little harder to quantity. Each had its unwanted effects on Sam too – he had to endure the spectacular mood swings of his hormonally challenged wife and the mutual and repeated devastation that was the consequence of each failure. Our feelings were amplified and, wherever we looked, we saw pregnant women.

We decided to take a break from the dizzying emotional roller coaster. This was certainly a time to clear our minds, mend our broken hearts and set aside our unfulfilled dreams, albeit temporarily.

We needed to recuperate emotionally and physically.

Most importantly, we had to focus on nurturing our marriage. We decided to have a twelve months, drug-free, holiday, in order to regain our physical, mental and spiritual strength. No needles, no pills, no pessaries, no scans. No more catching up on the latest magazine gossip in the specialist waiting room. No rituals, no praying and no worshipping of any pee-sticks. No expectations, no disappointments.

During our gap year, we had to ask ourselves some hard questions - most importantly, what would life be like without ever having a child?

This thought had constantly crossed my mind.

We would probably save a lot of money, because we wouldn't have to worry about bringing up a child or planning for his or her future. We could travel and go places without having to accommodate the needs of a small child.

I know there is a trend for professional couples to adopt animals instead of having children. I want to fast forward to thirty years from now and interview these couples. Has the thought of having a child ever come across their minds? If they had the power to turn back time, would they do anything differently? What is it like to be child free at this stage in life?

When we thought about that, what life would be like if we were unable to have you, Little One, we imagined our pampered pooch, Andy, going to doggie day care, accompanying us on plenty of road trips and having play dates with other dog socialites in town. Andy had his own tallboy filled with different outfits for different occasions. A special shelf was fitted in the pantry, at a dog-safety height, overcrowded with his favourite treats.

Every single corner of the house was a place for Andy to rest his paws. Sometimes I wondered, if only Andy could speak, what would he say? I hoped he would tell us that we would make great parents.

Although I was resting my body from the drugs, hormones and tests of conventional medicine, we did not rule out the possibility of alternative therapies.

"I don't want to push you or anything. Would you ever consider Chinese Medicine and acupuncture?" asked my husband, on his way home from work. "One of the nurses I worked with suggested it to someone nearby." I have always been quite stubborn when it comes to making any drastic changes in life. However, my husband was quite surprised with my response.

"Sure thing honey! I think it will be great to try alternative therapies. I have been doing some Internet research, I found a Chinese practitioner by the name of Dr Alice Gao. Is this the same person you are referring to?" I replied.

"Yes!" He was delighted that I had agreed so quickly.

Dr Alice Gao was a thinly built, modest middle-aged Chinese woman with more than twenty years of clinical experience both in China and Australia. The walls of the waiting room were covered with information on the Meridian Flow Chart and posters of some weird and funky looking tongues that reminded me of a certain performance at a recent music award ceremony.

I was pleased to read newspaper clippings, and some articles written by patients, with particular mention of certain IVF providers and Dr Alice Gao.

On another side of the room, there were many greeting cards and photos of cute looking babies, sleepy newborns, cuddly toddlers and autographed photos of some celebrities.

A strong herbal fragrance permeated the clinic, remaining me of my childhood. When I was growing up in Hong Kong, my grandmother used to collect herbs from the Chinese doctor. She would boil and reduce these herbs down to about a cupful of herbal soup. It was black in colour and tasted extremely bitter. My mother used to chase me around the house and force me to drink the herbal medicine. Who knew that, thirty-six years on, I would continue to follow my heritage and give Chinese medicine a try? This time though, in the hope of creating a little human being.

Since having a break from artificial reproductive treatments, my natural cycles were getting longer and longer. Aunt Flo used to visit every twenty-eight days, but gradually, the visits were becoming quite sparse – anywhere from thirty to forty-three days. I was experiencing terrible symptoms of night sweats, hot flushes and insomnia.

Dr Alice Gao was very attentive, caring and patient. To my surprise, Alice already had a good understanding of all of my previous IVF protocols. After taking a detailed clinical history, she explained the role and benefits of Chinese medicine and how this might help couples with infertility. She certainly answered many questions. I was so glad that we had found her.

In order to get a comprehensive understanding of my body's response during a natural cycle, Alice gave me specific instructions and plenty of homework. I had to chart my daily basal body temperature and to observe my cervical mucus around the time of ovulation.

I kept a diary of my mood swings, night sweats, hot flushes and insomnia. In addition, I was asked to do daily urine ovulation tests from day twelve of the cycle until I tested positive to a hormonal surge.

We understood that this was definitely not a quick fix or a get-me-pregnant-right-now treatment. Alice went on to explain that Chinese medicine worked in harmony with the body and therefore the response might be slower than the Western approach. She told me to persist and it would take about six months to regulate my natural hormonal response.

I started taking herbal medicine twice a day, in combination with weekly acupuncture sessions. Each week, the acupuncture points would be different.

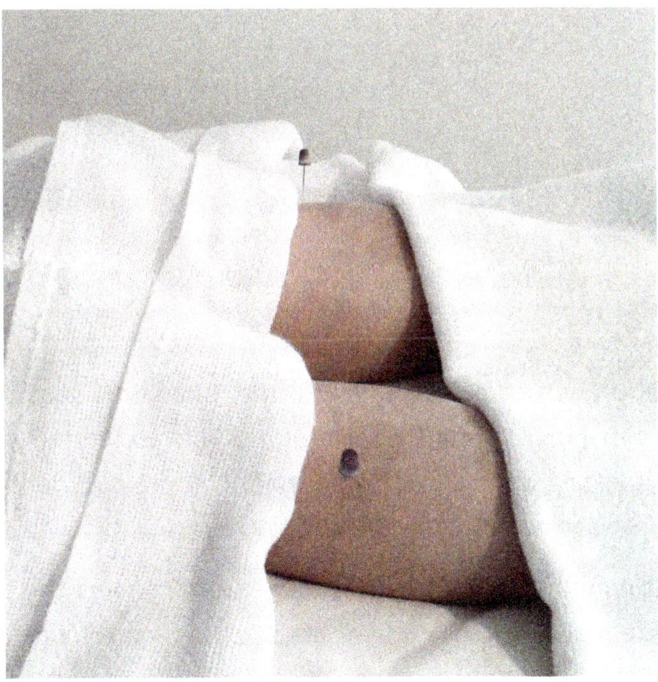

Various acupuncture points and moxibustion on my legs.

She used other treatment modalities too, such as heat cupping, Moxibustion and electrical stimulation. My favourite treatments were heat cupping and Moxibustion on the acupuncture points. For heat cupping, Alice used heat to create a vacuum effect on the aching and tense muscles on my shoulders, neck and back. This would help to increase blood flow to the area, aiding repair, healing and relaxing the muscles.

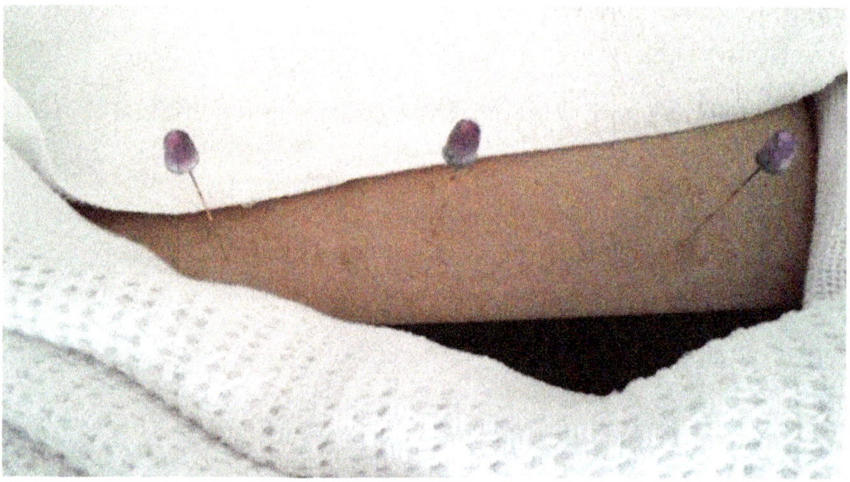

Acupuncture and Moxibustion on my belly. Very soothing.

Moxibustion was completely new to me. I had only seen it in the Jackie Chan movies when I was young. This technique involved carefully placing a burnt, dome-shaped, compressed herb on the top end of each acupuncture needle.

The heat would travel down the needles and conduct the thermal energy deeper into the target areas. The night following the treatments, I would have the best sleep and wake feeling refreshed the following day.

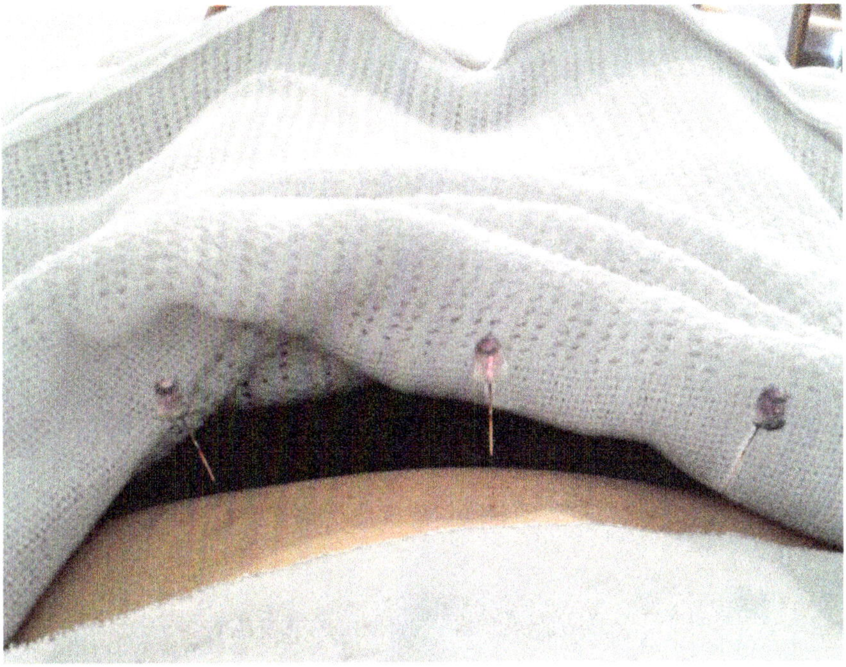

Acupuncture and Moxibustion on my belly. From the top view.

Dr Gao adjusted the herbal medicine every month depending on my body's response. To my amazement, within one month, my night sweats and hot flushes disappeared.

I started with a very low basal body temperature, along with some mid-cycle spotting that had been investigated in the past with no apparent cause.

Within two months, my basal body and post ovulation temperatures improved significantly. There was no further mid-cycle spotting and also the mood swings and irritable bowel symptoms reduced dramatically.

Alice advised us to listen to our bodies, introducing organic foods and essential fatty acids in our diets.

My husband diligently carried out some Internet research and found the best supplement combination for better quality "swimmers".

Alice also prescribed some herbal aphrodisiac for my husband; I named these "Chinese Viagra". He was instructed to take the medicine around my ovulation time. These little black pills worked wonders.

Chapter 10: Absolute Bliss

From: Sarah

Subject: Absolute Bliss

Date: 15 March 2013 5:32:34 pm AEDT

To: baby Babe

Dear baby Babe,

We have decided to take a year off to recover from the emotional toll and recent loses in life. Andy, your dog brother, had fallen very ill with pancreatitis. He lived for another six months but, late last year, he passed away peacefully from old age, in the comfort of our home. He was sixteen human years old. It was a very sad day.

Whilst we have been recuperating, we were given an opportunity to purchase a small beauty clinic business. I have been working at this clinic for four years, as an aesthetic doctor, and now the owner, Margarita, has decided that she will retire.

I am quite fortunate to have acquired the business with a smooth transition. I will continue my career as an aesthetic doctor, at least for now. I have since resigned as a General Practitioner, in late 2012. I do miss General Practice, however, the stress of running the business and recommencing another round of IVF was too much for me.

Wish me luck with the business. I promise, I will teach you everything I know.

Love, Sarah

During our break from the IVF treatments, we came across an opportunity to purchase a well-established beauty therapy business in Melbourne. Apart from being a General Practitioner, I had, by then, acquired special skills in cosmetic medicine and massage therapy, so I was able to provide exclusive services for clients at a beauty therapy clinic about 25 minutes drive from home.

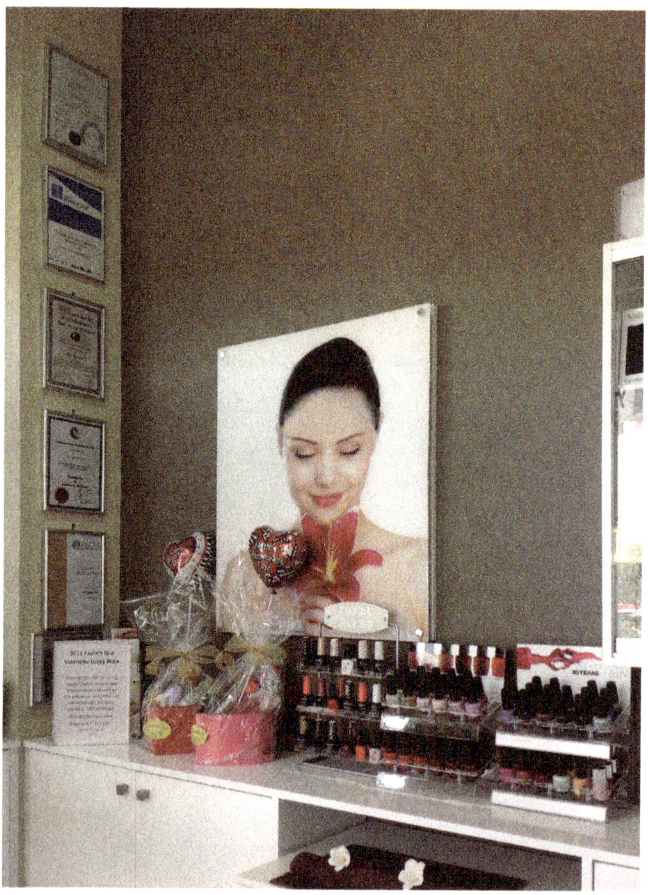

Reception area of the beauty clinic.

I loved my work there and was truly humbled by the whole experience, because the vendor, Margarita, was a much-adored Italian lady with so much passion, knowledge and experience. Her attitude to life and business was truly inspirational.

Just as I was looking for a business to buy, I discovered that she had put hers on the market, so that she could take a well-deserved retirement. We were both happy when I decided to buy the business. I did not enter the business blindly. I researched the area well in advance and had a good understanding of its demographics, average household income, median age group and ethnicity. It took six weeks to complete my thirty-two-page business plan. I wanted to prove to myself that success was possible with true determination.

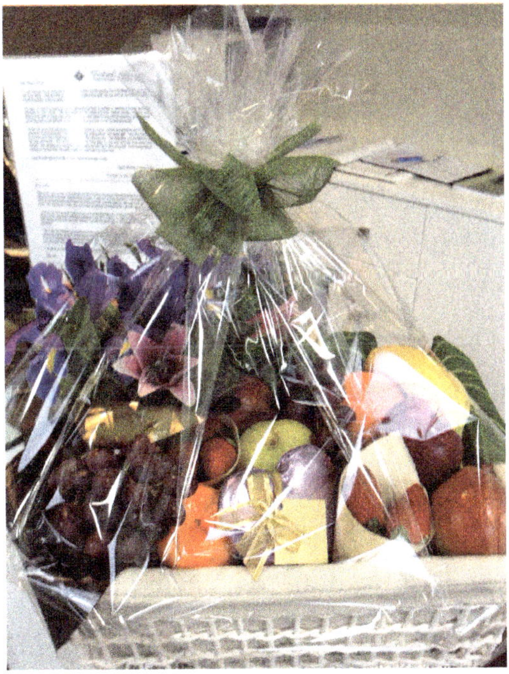

A beautiful hamper from the previous owner to congratulate myself as a new owner.

Margarita helped the transition enormously. I was so grateful for her guidance and pearls of wisdom.

Another useful source of information was LinkedIn. I joined various forums and followed a lot of leading experts in the field. I received daily updates on interesting and relevant articles on leadership, entrepreneurship and business management.

Having a father with many years of experience in a large-scale business management also helped, as we would throw new ideas at one another.

With Margarita's guidance, and the help of all the wonderful existing staff, the business grew steadily. It was a slow start, as we were like everyone else – weathering the global economic crisis. Also I took over at the start of a typical Melbourne winter. This was the quietest period in the beauty industry.

Having acquired a new loan and extra responsibilities, the first couple of months were difficult and I had to put in two hundred per cent effort with full dedication. Nevertheless, just a few months later, we enjoyed one of the busiest seasons in Christmas and New Year's.

I realized that I had to be patient. I must learn to walk before I can run. The vision was to provide the more desirable beauty services in the neighbourhood, with the best safety and hygiene of all. I felt rewarded by the opportunity to learn and nurture the business from its infancy.

For me, Absolute Bliss lived up to its name. It was so satisfying to be hands on in its advertising, marketing, growth and networking with other Cosmeceutical companies: it was extremely rewarding.

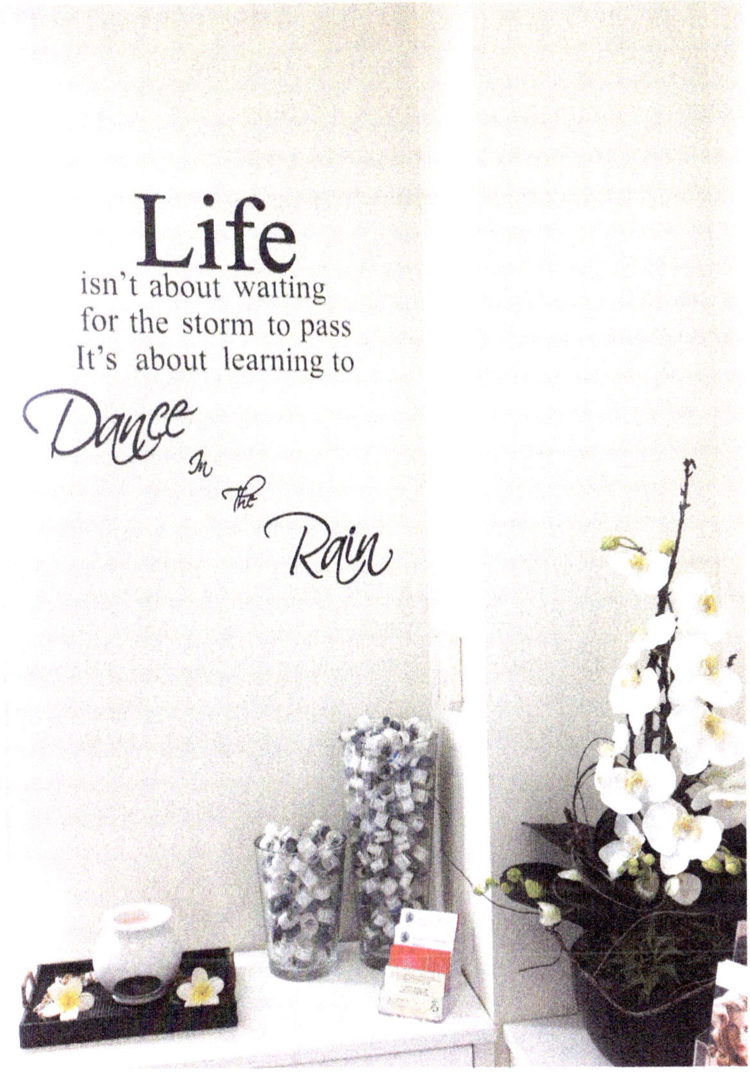
Life
isn't about waiting
for the storm to pass
It's about learning to
Dance
In
the
Rain

One of my favourite pieces of Wall Art from the clinic.
The flowers on the right are from my parents.

All the cushions I had made during the previous two-weeks' wait finally found a home at the beauty salon. Those beautiful scenic photos I took with my SLR camera were used in various advertising campaigns.

I had a newfound purpose in life, besides dealing with the repetitive torment of our IVF failures. Having a gap year from IVF treatments helped to build my confidence and self-esteem. As long as I put my mind and heart into something with absolute dedication and devotion, anything is possible. This gap year was a lifesaver for our marriage. We were able to spend more quality time together, to mend our wounds and to celebrate what we have overcome and achieved so far.

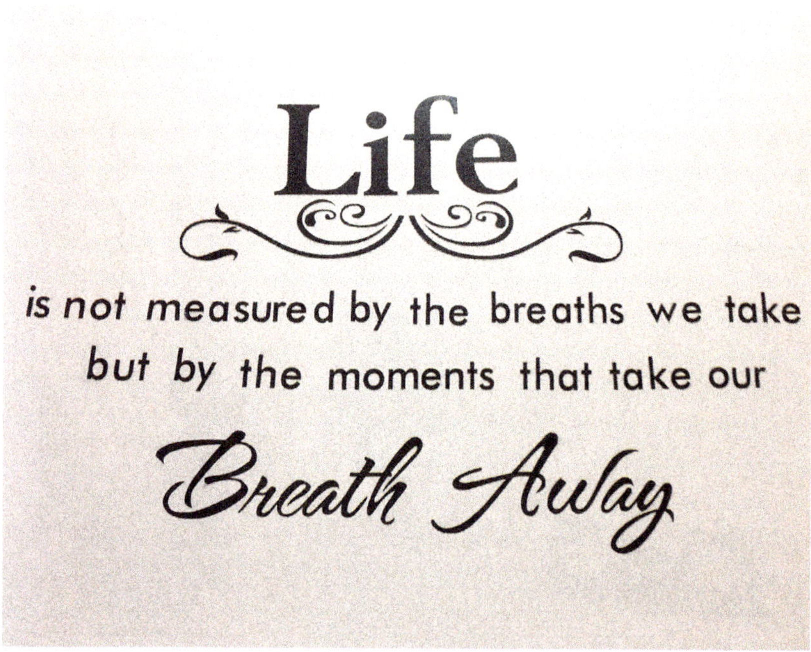

Wall Art near the pedicure area.

There was no point worrying about yesterday's failures and fears. We had learnt to count today's blessings and remain hopeful for tomorrow's events.

At the same time, I was still trying to balance General Practice and coping with our ailing geriatric dog, Andy. Andy had been in and out of the veterinary hospital. He had a frightening health scare earlier in 2012 and we almost lost him. Being a 16 year-old Silky-cross-Maltese, he required a lot of additional support. Due to my new work commitments, I felt terrible about leaving Andy at home for long periods of time. During the IVF cycles, Andy had been my faithful companion, especially when my husband was working long hours. When I was feeling sad and lonely, I took comfort in his loyal companionship. Whenever I looked into Andy's eyes, I knew that everything would be fine. Andy was my dog-child and he filled my void.

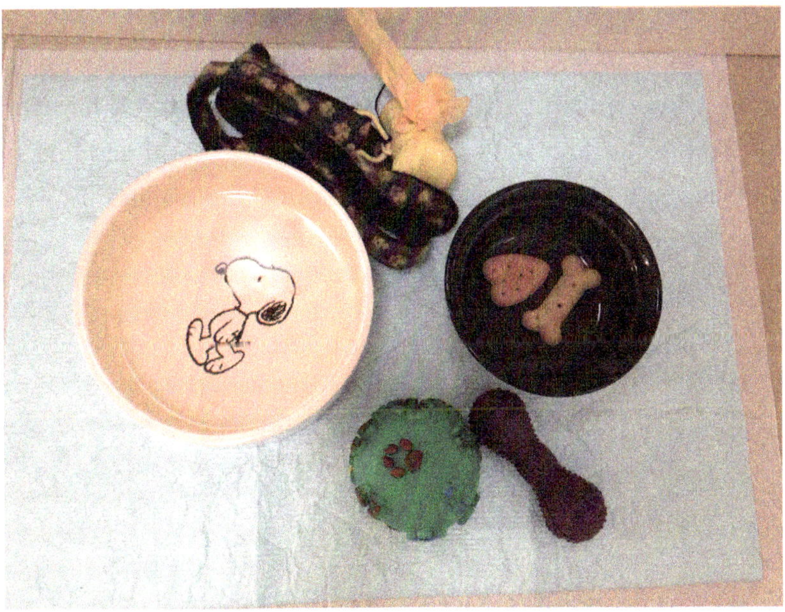

It took several weeks before I could find the strength to pack away Andy's belongings.

It was too much that the one bright, carefree soul in our home began to succumb.

Andy, our beautiful little dog, was aging before our eyes. In late September 2012, his now geriatric little body was clearly in distress. We raced him to the vet, but he deteriorated very rapidly. I cut back on my working hours to spend as much time with him as I could, but nothing could stop his deterioration.

On 4 October, Andy finally left this world.

I woke up early that morning and found him sleeping soundly in his bed. As I went to give him a cuddle, he woke up and stared at me with his innocent but tired eyes. We went for a very short stroll, just up to my next-door neighbour's front yard, before he got too tired. I carried him home and I could sense that this might be his last, final walk. I bathed him in warm water and blow-dried his coat whilst massaging his arthritic legs.

He really enjoyed his bath, as the warm water offered him some relief from pain, and took the weight off his legs. I cuddled him and placed him on my chest for the rest of the morning.

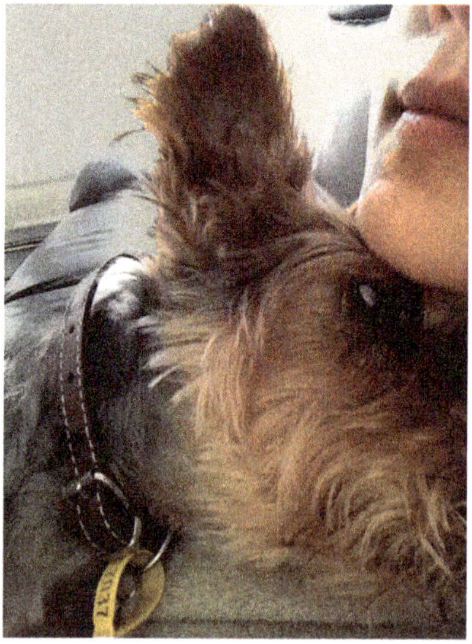

He was exhausted, with shallow breathing, and I could feel him slipping away. I was glad to be able to embrace him and make him feel my love in his final moments. He passed away peacefully, in the comfort of his favourite pillow, a few hours later, a few days before our sixth wedding anniversary.

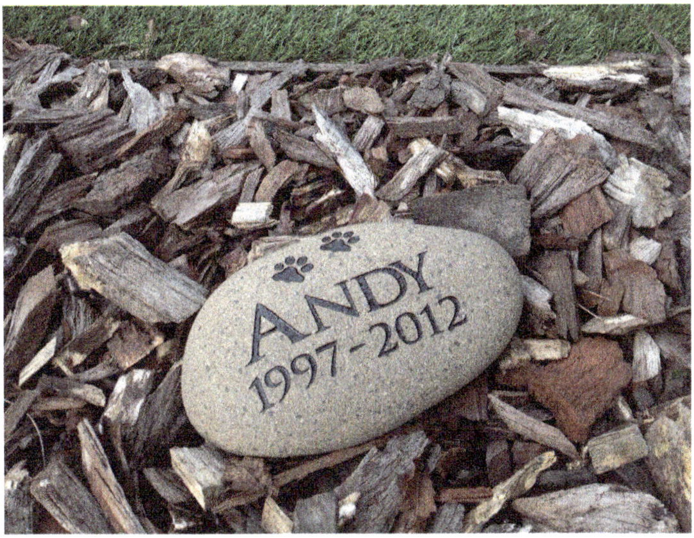

We were shattered. He had been our precious playmate and comfort, who licked the tears away when we couldn't bear the losses we were handed. You would have loved him, baby. And he would have loved you.

Some friends trivialised our loss. Little did they know how hard we had been battling infertility and how losing our Andy brought back all the memories of failed IVF attempts and underlined our childlessness. Our wedding anniversary came and went without celebration that year. What was there to celebrate?

I was truly grateful for what Andy had given us, a chance to provide unconditional love and an opportunity to receive love in return. After Andy's passing, I decided to take an indefinite leave from general practice. The new business, the recent loss of a beloved dog and the prospect of, perhaps, recommencing the IVF treatments, were the main reasons of dropping the General Practice sessions, but also, and ironically, I specialized in women's health and pregnancy care.

Every pregnant woman that came through the door was a constant reminder of my childless state. I would found myself bursting into tears between the consultations. I realized there was only one option. I resigned. Two weeks before my last day, a nurse from Monash IVF visited my clinic to speak about the work being done at Monash. I spoke with her after the session and took note of her name. I was already under Melbourne IVF, but who knew what the future held? I took her card and filed it away.

The memory of my last general practice patient was crystal clear. A university student presented with her mother for advice about an unplanned pregnancy. The entire consultation was emotionally charged. Both the mother and daughter expressed a combination of anger, denial, guilt and sadness within the time frame of a standard consultation.

This was the ultimate test. At the end of the consultation, I was choking back my tears when the patient asked me, "what would you do doctor, if you were in my position?"

Fortunately, they prepare you in medical school for just such a question. "It doesn't matter what I would do, because you're not me and I'm not you."

This answer might not have completely satisfied her, but it satisfied my need to remain true to the ethical stance every doctor must take. I switched off my humanity button, to ensure that my advice was not clouded by my own personal experience. Deep down inside, my heart was screaming at my head.

This was just too hard. I found that, almost through necessity, I had begun to distance myself emotionally from everyone, including my patients. Resignation had been the right decision, so on 17 November 2012, I walked out of my clinic, and my life as a general practitioner, unsure if I would ever pick up my stethoscope again.

I buried myself in my work and it took a very long time before I could finish the day without shredding a single tear.

Little One, you will find that sometimes in life, things happen for a reason. Quite often these reasons are unknown to us at the time and their blessings are not available to us until we view them in retrospect.

Two months into my Absolute Bliss management, one of my permanent, full time staff sustained a horrific injury at home. She had multiple lacerations in her arms, lower body and legs. I was devastated to learn of her injuries, because she was such a beautiful young woman, with so much potential.

She was a devoted worker and adored by our staff and clients. I kept in touch with her family to keep track of her progress and recovery. Having a medical background was helpful in understanding the nature of her injuries and the type of operations that she underwent. Based on this, I was able to draw some assumptions and predict her likelihood of returning to work.

I had the privilege of working with this young lady for a few months prior to acquiring the business. Her professionalism and the way that she presented herself were immaculate. Since this was not a WorkCover related injury, as an employer, it was not my responsibility to offer a return to work plan.

However, my instincts motivated and inspired me to help this staff member. My manager was an absolutely fantastic woman. Together, we were able to draw up a special return to work plan for her. As I had had a lot of experience in dealing with WorkCover patients in general practice, we were able to tailor a special plan for her.

Included in my philosophies in life are: to recognize the potentials in everyone, have a bit of faith and give second chances after taking a well-measured and calculated risk.

Similar to IVF treatments, we recognized the possibility of failure, however, we chose to take a leap of faith against all measured risks. It was a decision based on my medical knowledge and gut instincts.

Weeks and months passed by and I could not believe my eyes. Not only did she defy all odds, she turned out to be one of my best employees. With the help of my manager, this young woman blossomed under our well-structured return to work plan.

She was hard working, loyal and devoted to her work, colleagues and clients. She genuinely loved coming to work every day and enjoyed every moment of it. It was most rewarding to see such a positive engagement from her. I was grateful for her return to part time work after several months of rehabilitation.

One day, the topic of compassion came up in our conversation. To my surprise, she commented, "Sarah, I think you are the most compassionate person I have ever met."

I believed her words were genuine and not spoken simply because I was her boss. She spoke while seeing me eye to eye as an equal. I was touched. I thanked her humbly and quickly looked away as happy tears flooded my eyes.

I might have given up the stethoscope but perhaps there were still opportunities for me to heal.

Having a gap year from IVF treatments, a business to run and the positive feedback from people like this young woman, had a big impact on building my confidence and self-esteem.

I had a newfound purpose in my life that had, until then, been racked by the torment of repeated IVF failures. It brought new strength to our marriage as well. We had gradually and cautiously let go of the pain and fear and simply filled the year with fun.

We bought bikes and cycled; we dined out; we went to the movies and the driving range (turns out golf is not my greatest skill). Every weekend we just did as we pleased - it was all about spontaneity.

It mended wounds and celebrated what we had overcome to this point and what we had achieved.

This was a precious year that I would never regret. Perhaps it meant delaying our meeting with you, but I was confident that you would have happier, closer parents should that day ever arrive.

And so, our year of rest and relaxation over, we began to turn our minds back towards the IVF maw.

Chapter 11: Moving Forward

From: Sarah

Subject: Next round at Monash

Date: 15 March 2013 8:32:34 pm AEDT

To: baby Babe

Dear baby Babe,

We have decided to try our very best this year. No matter how many cycles, I am determined to fall pregnant. We both feel that we are ready to be parents and hope that, one day, you will come into our lives.

Monash IVF has been absolutely fantastic. I had surgery a few weeks ago and found out that, indeed, I had endometriosis. So, that makes sense as to why we have had trouble conceiving. I wish that I had found out earlier.

We are ready for a fresh new start.

Love, Sarah

Time had passed and wounds had healed, although imperfectly, by early 2013, so it was up battle gears to make another attempt. This time, we moved in a different direction. I recalled the IVF nurse, from Monash IVF, who had visited my general practice before I resigned and introduced Monash IVF services to all of our staff. I had been given the opportunity to ask questions and compared the success rates across the top IVF providers in town. There were similarities, and some distinct differences, in Monash's IVF philosophies and techniques from those I had been using. I had been intrigued. At the end of the meeting, I'd had a private conversation with the nurse. She appreciated that I had shared my experience and encouraged me to meet and speak to the Director of Monash IVF, Dr Lynn Burmeister.

It was time we shook things up, and tried something new, so I decided to follow her suggestion. It was not easy getting an appointment with Dr Burmeister. She was considered to be a guru and pioneer in artificial reproductive treatments in Melbourne, so women like me flocked to her door. Whenever her name was mentioned alongside celebrities, many of whom had finally had successful IVF births, Dr Burmeister's website would crash instantly, from so many people wanting to know more.

The first available appointment with her was three months away and I put myself down on a waiting list should any patients cancel at the last minute. In the meantime, I contacted Monash IVF to explain that I was already an IVF patient with a different provider. Fortunately, our legal documents were still valid, so we did not have to endure new police and working with children checks. However, we were still required to go through a compulsory counselling session with the new provider.

Saturday appointments were hard to come by, for counselling sessions, because many couples worked full time. There was usually a six months wait. Fortunately, we were lucky, because a couple cancelled and we were seen within a fortnight.

All of the necessary paperwork was done during the time I waited to see Dr Burmeister. When my day finally arrived, I gathered all of my previous treatment protocols, blood tests and ultrasound reports and set out.

The specialist's room was designed to her personal taste and style. One side of the wall was covered with hundreds of happy baby photos, in all shapes and sizes; most of them were milk drunk some way or the other. On the other side of the wall was a large heart shape decoration, made out of knitted green bamboo straws. In between, the phones were going nonstop, and the receptionist answered with a most calming and professional manner.

Dr Lynn Burmeister was a very tall, slim and fashionable woman. She had long red hair with curled ends giving it a soft, wavy, stylish look. Her soft and intelligent blue eyes immediately reassured me that everything would be fine. I presented all the details of the previous antagonist cycles to her. She recommended a down regulation cycle (in which ovulation is supressed) and a "clean up" procedure prior to commencement of this new cycle. A "clean up" would involve a hysteroscopy (a camera to look into the cavity of the uterus) via dilatation, followed by curettage (scraping out) of the uterus. She explained that there is evidence to suggest that doing this, prior to commencing artificial reproductive treatments, increased the chance of success.

There was something else. I'd had a rather odd cycle a few months before this consultation. It was on Christmas Day that I'd had period pains much worse than I'd ever experienced before. They were so bad that a combination of paracetamol and ibuprofen barely touched them. After cooking a four-course Christmas dinner, I'd excused myself to lie down and rest, in the bedroom, for the rest of the evening. The pain was excruciating. I could hardly catch my breath. I knew I was definitely not pregnant, and again wondered if I could be suffering from endometriosis. So in addition to having this clean up procedure, she proposed that I have a laparoscopy done at the same time. Since the surgery was going to be performed under general anaesthetic, I wanted to exclude other sinister conditions, which might have caused that severe period pain episode.

Once again, waiting to undergo surgery and shivering inside my thin patient gown. The blood pressure cuff on my right arm inflated. The anaesthetist carefully examined my left hand so he could find that much-pierced vein. I concentrated on the low-flow oxygen rustling through the mask.

"Don't you worry, we will look after you", said Dr Burmeister as she gave me a gentle stroke on my right shoulder.

"Just relax and count to ten. I am going to give you some medicine to help you to sleep," my anaesthetist said as he squirted some cold white Propofol into the intravenous line. I briefly thought of Propofol's association with the late King of Pop, Michael Jackson.

I think I had a coughing fit before I fell asleep. The room was getting darker and I was seeing double. I found myself drifting away so quickly I did not even have the chance to count past five.

Why do heat packs only come in the shape of a rectangle? I was kindly given a large heat pack to settle the post-operative pain. If it was designed by a woman, it would certainly be a fashionable black and in the shape of a half doughnut or V-shaped so as to better accommodate our needs. As I placed the warm pack on my lower abdomen, its ends stuck out, heating below my groin onto my upper thighs. No matter how I placed it, there was heat wastage. I must patent my half-doughnut design one day. Still, I appreciated the small act of care and kindness from the person who gave me this thing – the heat pack dulled the stabbing pain before it overwhelmed me.

Dr Burmeister came to visit me in the recovery room. She confirmed that I had moderate endometriosis and adenomyosis (abnormal tissue found within the uterine wall).

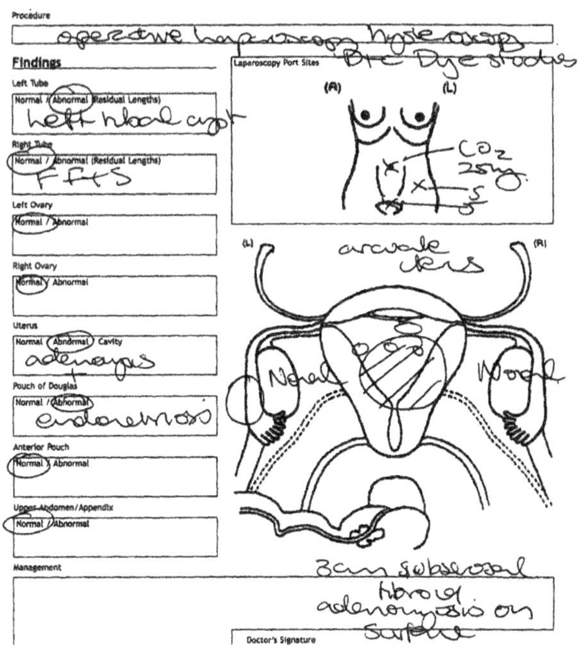

My operative notes.

When they performed the dye test, the left tube seemed to be blocked, but she said that the occlusion could have been the result of spasm. She was quite confident that the tubes looked fine on laparoscopic view. She considered our chances of success to be quite high.

Over the next few days, I developed a fever, gastritis from not being able to stomach any food, and diarrhoea from the antibiotics, despite taking regular probiotics. I was lucky that I had taken two weeks off work. On the bright side, it must have been a very good "clean up" as I had also lost a few kilos.

Chapter 12: Survival of the Fittest

From: Sarah

Subject: hormone overdrive

Date: 17 March 2013 11:14:57 am AEDT

To: baby Babe

Dear baby Babe,

I had the last injection, the Trigger injection (to release the eggs from the follicles) at 8:30 pm last night. This morning, I have woken up with less back pain, but feeling really tired, super emotional and hormonal today. I feel sorry for your dad and everyone else around me. I think everything is working at overdrive. It will soon be over.

The egg collection is scheduled tomorrow at 8:30 am and I have to arrive at the day surgery at 7 am for admission.

Let's hope everything will go smoothly.

I am ready. We will survive.

Love, Sarah

The theory behind the Down Regulation cycle is similar to rebooting a computer. The thinking behind it is that by suppressing the Luteinising Hormone, which stimulates ovulation, for a monthly cycle, then, the following month, stimulating ovulation, the ovaries will hopefully respond by improving egg quantity.

I met my IVF nurse, Charlotte, for the first time. She explained the entire stimulated cycle with very clear written instructions. The dates, times and different types of medications were all explained in detail.

She also discussed the timeline for scans, blood tests, egg pick up and embryo transfer. I was impressed by, and grateful for, the co-ordination of the schedule of appointments.

This really helped to alleviate the stress of having to fit everything in with my working schedule. Best of all, she brought along all the IVF medications in a bag. I remembered, from previous treatments, that some of the medications must be kept refrigerated, so I had brought along my esky, loaded with icepacks. I was prepared and more than ready.

In a nutshell, I had to take the contraceptive pill for twenty-one days, followed by a twice daily dose of a nasal spray. Both of these medications would suppress the ovarian function and produce transient menopausal side effects.

Wonderful! Your poor father would have to deal with my crazy hormones again. Hopefully, this time, the side effects would be short-lived, because, with them, I would not be the most popular person around, at least for a while.

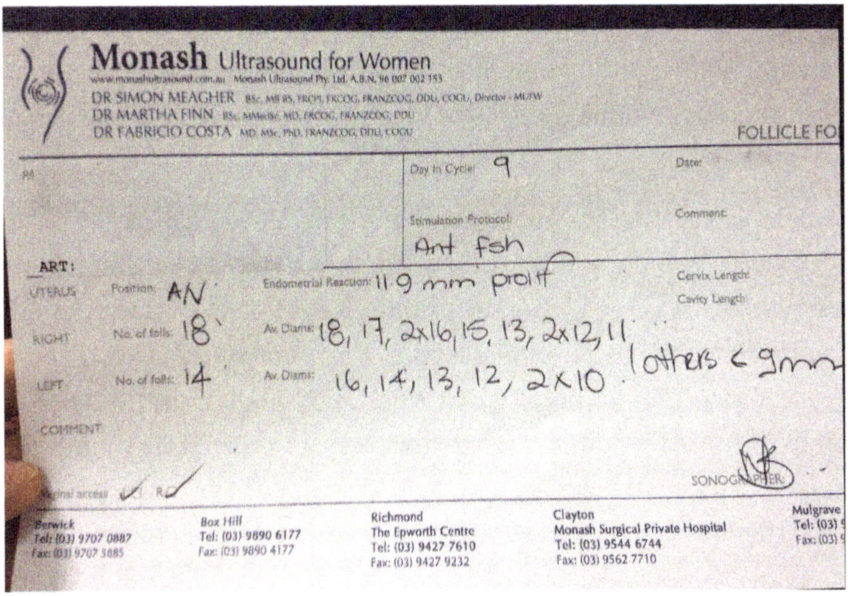

Monash Ultrasound for Women
www.monashultrasound.com.au Monash Ultrasound Pty. Ltd. A.B.N. 96 007 002 153
DR SIMON MEAGHER
DR MARTHA FINN
DR FABRICIO COSTA
FOLLICLE FO

Day in Cycle: 9
Date:
Stimulation Protocol: Ant fsh
Comment:

ART:
UTERUS Position: AN Endometrial Reaction: 11.9 mm prolif
Cervix Length:
Cavity Length:
RIGHT No. of folls: 18 Av. Diams: 18, 17, 2x16, 15, 13, 2x12, 11
LEFT No. of folls: 14 Av. Diams: 16, 14, 13, 12, 2x10 / others < 9mm
COMMENT:
SONOGRAPHER:

Berwick Tel: (03) 9707 0887 Fax: (03) 9707 5885
Box Hill Tel: (03) 9890 6177 Fax: (03) 9890 4177
Richmond The Epworth Centre Tel: (03) 9427 7610 Fax: (03) 9427 9232
Clayton Monash Surgical Private Hospital Tel: (03) 9544 6744 Fax: (03) 9562 7710
Mulgrave

My internal pelvic ultrasound report. Lots of follicles!!

We collected seventeen eggs as a result of this down regulation cycle. Out of these eggs, six fertilized, but only three embryos survived to day five.

One was used for the immediate fresh transfer and the other two were to be frozen for later use. The main differences with this cycle were threefold: a special liquid medium was used to select the best quality sperms for fertilization; secondly, day-five embryos were used for transfers instead of day-three embryos, thereby transferring the fittest of all; thirdly, the transfer itself was performed under ultrasound guidance.

In order to locate the best position for the transfer, a full bladder was required to ensure a better view under ultrasound guidance. How difficult was it to swallow two litres of water in an hour? Very.

With a small bladder capacity, I ended up having to go to the bathroom several times before the procedure, then refilling it to ensure an appropriately full bladder. It was like a water drinking marathon.

Luckily, I was the first patient of the day. I was called into the procedure room at eight-thirty on the dot. Inside the room, everything was, of course, immaculately clean and super-sanitized, with that unmistakable hospital smell. I was first greeted by the embryologist, who had been babysitting our embryo for a few days prior to this transfer. She showed me an enlarged image of the embryo and described it briefly stating it was the best quality out of the three. At last, I could finally visualize the embryo, face to face. *'My Preccccious!!'* I was in awe.

Oh my goodness, that was some cold jelly on my belly. As the doctor was holding the sterile speculum inside Miss V, the nurse pressed the ultrasound probe firmly over my bladder. *'No! YOU try relaxing on a full bladder when people are poking on the bladder!'* Thankfully, I said it to myself.

It was difficult to relax. *'Don't pee, please don't pee. Not here, not now. Don't you dare embarrass yourself in front of your colleagues'*, lectured the doctor-voice inside my head. This was a newfound meaning of 'peer pressure'.

The actual transfer took less than five minutes but it was probably the longest five minutes of the entire IVF cycle. I was so embarrassed and I didn't know where to look except at the ceiling. What did other women talk about during such an undignified procedure? The Masterchef series? The Ellen Show? The weather? The football? Politics?

Finally, I mentioned something about the recent crazy weather as we had been having extreme hot and cold days. Everyone nodded quickly, perhaps also wanting to break the seemingly impenetrable ice. *'Maybe I should have got a Brazilian XXX a few days ago,'* I thought to myself.

Once the ideal position for transfer was located, the doctor informed the embryologist that he was ready for the embryo transfer. The precious cargo was carried in, from the mini laboratory adjacent to the procedure room. We all held our breaths in anticipation of the most important thing alive, with the price tag of $10,000, yet invisible to any naked eye. At the end of the procedure, the nurse reminded me to start the progesterone pessary at night. This was to continue until the day of the blood test.

I was not feeling well. Twenty-four hours after the transfer, I developed a shocking headache and a fever of 38 degrees Celsius (100.4 degrees Fahrenheit). I had the usual cramps and had been running to the bathroom with some urinary frequency.

The fever settled after a dose of paracetamol and a good night's rest. What was that about? I wondered.

Four days later, I woke up during the night to find that I had had some bleeding. Between the time of leaving a voicemail, for my nurse to get when she arrived at work in the morning, to the time she returned my call a few short hours later, Aunt Flo had arrived. I was devastated. Neither my nurse, Dr Gao or I had heard of anyone bleeding so early after the transfer. Despite this, I was instructed to continue with the vaginal progesterone pessaries every night and wait for the blood test.

Raging Aunt Flo was relentless. She stayed for the next seven, miserable days. The blood test confirmed what we already knew: a negative pregnancy. Dr Gao then used acupuncture and Moxibustion to try relieving my stress, tension and pain. I was grateful that she offered me extra time during the treatment, in order to facilitate my recovery and healing. I lay half naked and exposed with acupuncture needles embedded in points all over my body, but the incense rising from the Moxibustion calmed my fidgety nerves.

The warmth of the Moxibustion travelled deep into my lower abdomen. I was comforted by the intensity of this heat. A sense of healing infiltrated every crevice and emptiness within this exhausted body of mine. The sound of teardrops seemed amplified by the silence. Trickle. Trickle. Trickle. I could not reach them. My hands were pinned down.

What happened to my precious? Why didn't it stay? Why did I bleed so early? Was my womb so hostile? Was it the fever? What the?

Chapter 13: Steroid Mania and Injections Galore

From: Sarah

Subject: Update

Date: 27 March 2013 4:09:19 pm AEDT

To: baby Babe

The fresh embryo transfer happened on Sat the 23rd March 2013.

Today is day 4-post transfer but, unfortunately, I experienced a lot of cramps upon waking up this morning and I started to bleed. Initially it was a dark cherry colour in two lots of 50-cent piece sized, but as the day has gone by, it got brighter and brighter and it's looking more like a normal Aunt Flo (period).

I have called the nurse and she said it is rather uncommon for it to happen. I will have to continue with the progesterone pessary until the day of the blood test on next Wednesday morning.

It is not looking good. We have only got TWO frosties left. So, hopefully one of them will be you.

Happy Easter. I was hoping for an Easter miracle, never mind!

I know it will happen.

Love, Sarah

"I want you to page me if you bleed within the first few days after the next transfer. This is very unusual." Dr Lynn Burmeister was alarmed at what happened. "That was a very nice embryo and I am sorry that we couldn't get you pregnant."

She went on to explain that she was going to put me on a special protocol, The Bondi Protocol. A Sydney IVF doctor working in Bondi first introduced this very specific treatment plan and it worked for a lot of women with issues of high immunity and implantation failure. There are cells known as Natural Killers (NK) cells that would normally help to fight viruses and bacteria in the body. However, in certain women, these levels are particularly high and, theoretically, might mistakenly think that the embryo, which obtained half of its genetic material from the husband, was foreign to the body.

HISTOPATHOLOGY OF BIOPSY MATERIAL

CLINICAL NOTES:
Endometrial biopsy. Histology and NK cells.
MACROSCOPIC DESCRIPTION:
Labelled with patients details only - a scant amount of haemorrhagic tissue 10mm x 6mm x 1mm in aggregate dimension. A1. (SW/nt/dp)
MICROSCOPIC DESCRIPTION:
The biopsy includes a few tiny fragments of endometrium in which there are inactive tubular glands separated by abundant stroma. There is no evidence of chronic endometritis, atypical hyperplasia or malignancy. Immunoperoxidase staining for CD56, a marker of natural killer cells, shows moderate numbers of stromal cells with positive staining at a rate of the order of 15 cells per high power field, but only 2 high power fields of tissue are available for assessment.
DIAGNOSIS:
ENDOMETRIAL BIOPSY - SCANTY INACTIVE ENDOMETRIUM. NATURAL KILLER CELLS ARE DEMONSTRATED AT A RATE OF THE ORDER OF 15 CELLS PER HIGH POWER FIELD.

My endometrial (uterine lining) biopsy report.

When I thought about it, I realised that I actually don't get sick easily. Being exposed to ill patients over the years, with coughs and colds, might have helped to build a stronger immune system. Who knew this might one day be detrimental to my natural fertility?

I was sick for two straight weeks a few years ago, but that was probably the only time I had been that truly unwell. I survived the swine flu pandemic unscathed.

The Bondi protocol involved taking a combination of low dose prednisolone, antibiotics and clexane – an anticoagulant delivered via injection. Great! More drugs and more injections and just two frosty embryos left. I prayed that at least one of them would decide to stick around a bit longer.

For a Frozen Embryo Transfer (FET) cycle, the timing of my ovulation was crucial. Precision was the key.

Since the most recent stimulation cycle, my previous record had been broken, now my longest ever recorded natural cycle was forty-four days. Normally, most women have regular twenty-one to twenty-eight day cycles. This meant that the optimal moment for transfer was even harder to determine in me.

Charlotte explained that the urine ovulation kits might not be as accurate as the FET needed. "I am sorry Sarah, but we will have to get you to do a blood test every second day, starting on day twelve of your cycle."

The blood tests would indicate early changes in the hormone levels and, therefore, they would be able to pinpoint the big 'O' - ovulation day. Once the day was set, a blastocyst (also known as the day-five embryo) would be prepared in the laboratory to make its journey home. This would be done on the fifth day after ovulation.

Thank goodness for the one and only large, blood-donating vein in my left arm. This poor fella had to be pricked every other day.

The nurses each made their unique signatures by encircling the vein. I would be suspicious too if anyone had track marks on their veins.

Twelve! Due to a rather delayed ovulation, I endured twelve blood tests over two long weeks, not to mention waking up before six every morning, and rushing through the peak hour traffic, in order to make it in time for the morning blood collection. Luckily, I don't suffer from belonephobia (fear of sharp things, especially needles). Breathe, Sarah. Breathe. Stop complaining. This blood-letting is a small sacrifice to make.

I had been on steroids for a week, and I had not noticed anything different, until my manager mentioned that I had been particularly "excitable" and "talkative".

Those were her exact words. My husband commented that he could not follow my conversations, as I was having slightly pressured speech with a flight of ideas. *'That's rubbish'*, I thought to myself. I might have been running out of breath whenever I was having a decent conversation with someone, anyone. I didn't mind – I was as happy as Larry. The only problem was that I could not sleep.

'Go to bed. It's two in the morning, why can't I fall asleep?' I was tossing and turning around. Blankets on; blankets off. I looked at my iPhone and checked my Facebook updates. I played Candy Crash, on silent mode of course, until I had no more candy lives left. I would have to wait another twenty minutes before I could play again. I also used the iPad before moving on to the computer in the study room. *'I must resist the temptation. I have to go to bed. Someone has to get up to go to work.'*

I was starting to get angry with myself.

Surprised by how little sleep I could get by on, I was only sleeping three to four hours per night. Two weeks later, my body finally waved the little white flag and succumbed to the effects of chronic fatigue.

I was in burnt-out mode, tired and losing my marbles. It got worse after the transfer, because by then I was suffering from the side effects of a high dose of progesterone.

Has anyone seen my favourite writing pen? I was just using it an hour ago. Can someone please explain to me what is the TV remote doing in the fridge? Some silly person must have been so hungry that she forgot about the remote whilst rummaging for food. What is that burnt smell? I burnt my sunny-side-up egg! I don't remember making that this morning. Is this early dementia setting in?

I finally resorted to having little yellow post it notes all over my computer, the fridge door and the entire house. Not a pretty look. I hoped that this would be short-lived and not get passed onto the next generation.

19 June, 2013: I arrived at the day surgery clinic on time for the long awaited transfer. When the doors of the lift opened, I thought I had stumbled into a childcare centre. Twins! There was a set of twins screaming and playing loudly with their toys in the very same waiting area.

Their father was busy 'Skyping' a relative via his iphone and you could hear a woman baby-talking in a foreign language to these toddlers.

It went on for almost an hour. There were a lot of unfriendly stares, as the room was full and packed with women having embryo transfers.

Overly sensitive and upset, partly due to my hormones, I found myself hiding behind a row of chairs, cursing inside my head. Surely, people ought to be more considerate.

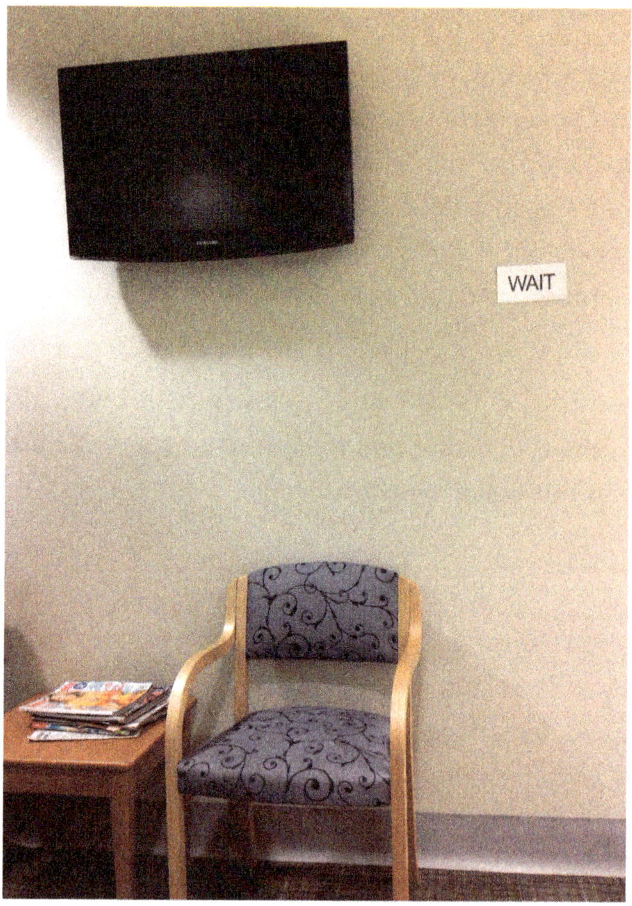

My life seemed to be a waiting game.

This was a waiting room in a fertility centre; full of desperate couples anxiously waiting for an elective, expensive and uncomfortable procedure. Why am I thinking like this? I am usually a much more tolerant person.

My – our – eighth transfer. Lucky eight, right? An hour had passed; I was still waiting. I walked awkwardly to the reception area to check the progress of the queue.

As this transfer was to be done under ultrasound guidance, my full bladder was screaming at me, it wanted to explode.

Finally, after a few words of introduction, prodding and poking, the embryo was transferred back home. I quickly made my way to see Dr Gao for the post transfer acupuncture. This was pretty much my routine.

To pee or not to pee on a stick? Two weeks wait was up; I finally folded and took a home pregnancy test.

My breasts were a little more tender than usual, especially the right side. It must be my imagination, as the right breast was a bit lumpy and sore. Is this my lucky day today?

One line. Five minutes later? One single line.

No matter how long I waited; no matter how I flipped and rotated the stick in and out of the light, it was one single blue line. Negative. Disappointed.

I arrived on time for work, after driving through the heavy peak hour traffic from the pathology centre. It was around lunchtime when I started to bleed. It was over. Feeling rather emotional and tearful, I kept myself busy and soldiered on until another day was gone, done and dusted.

I felt sorry for the nurse who called and confirmed yet another negative pregnancy test. I knew how tough it was to repeatedly give bad news.

Chapter 14: Road Block and Detour

From: Sarah

Subject: Not looking good

Date: 26 June 2013 02:16:27 PM AEST

To: baby Babe

Dear baby Babe,

It is not looking good. What else do I have to do to?

I am just so frustrated. I know I haven't done anything wrong but I feel like a complete failure and this must be some sort of punishment.

If this cycle doesn't work, I know the problem lies within me. I am scared.

Love, Sarah

After a few months of rest, we decided to push on and continue with our last frozen embryo.

'Ouch. What the? This is new.' The week before the scheduled transfer I noted that the lumpiness on the right side of my breast had not resolved, despite me being off all of the medications. This painful lump had doubled in size since the last embryo transfer.

I freaked. Out of panic and desperation, I organized an ultrasound for the following day.

For the first time, I was greeted by warmed and peppermint-scented ultrasound gel. Little things mattered most. It was certainly a big contrast to the freezing cold gels they used during the embryo transfers.

As the sonographer was running the ultrasound probe up and down my right breast, I kept a curious eye on the ultrasound screen. Bingo. There it was! The sonographer located an oval lesion with a shadow inside it.

A stern doctor-voice in my head spoke to me calmly: *'It is probably just another benign breast lump. Considering the amount of hormones you are taking, it's not surprising that the breast tissue has proliferated. Don't worry about it!'*

It was drowned out by the anxious patient-voice in my head:

'Oh my goodness! This is a rapidly growing breast tissue. You have been on high doses of hormone agents for a few years. You know very well that there is a family history of breast cancer. If this is truly the 'C-word', this will be the end of your IVF journey, the end of everything. Go and see someone, Stat!'

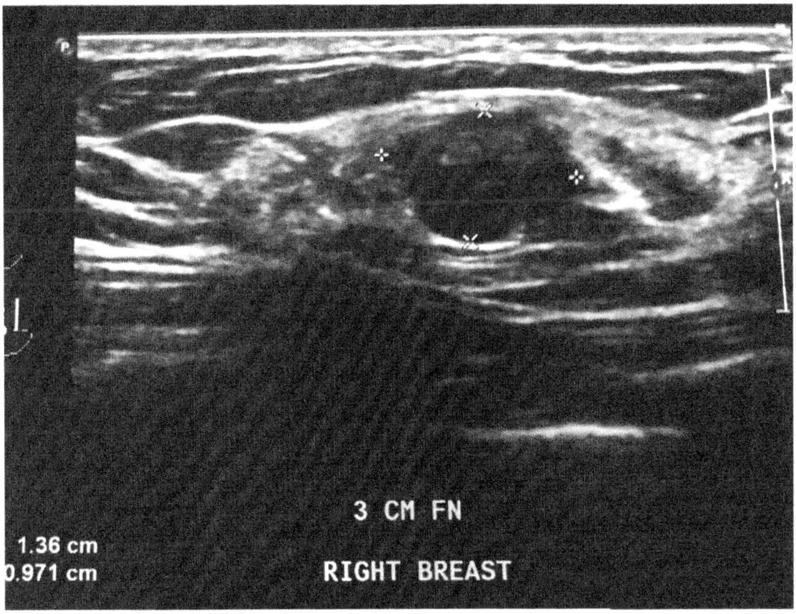

New lesion noted on my right breast

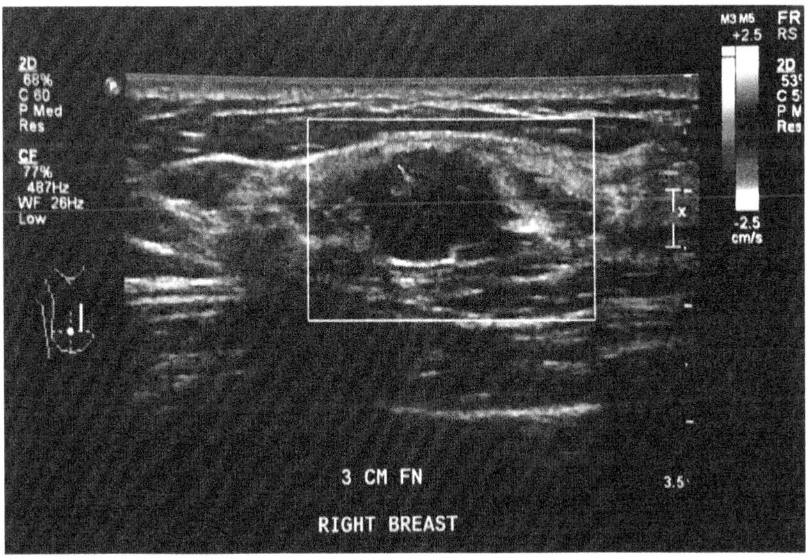

The doctor-voice was overwhelmingly unsympathetic and dismissive: *'Get a grip of yourself! You are a medical doctor and you should know better. Stop wasting time and get on with the program.'*

But my patient-voice was having none of that: *'Don't listen to her! It is normal to feel scared and doubtful, to be anxious and worried. You are only human. We have to take this seriously. If you don't take charge of looking after yourself, no one can do that for you.'*

I was trying not to scream out loud, to silence the voices in my head. The final embryo transfer was scheduled for one week's time. This was a most unwelcome detour and unnecessary stress.

Standing by the car door outside the imaging centre, I panicked and called your father. Once again, the poor guy had been anxiously waiting by the phone at work all day. He recommended contacting the MBU, Melbourne Breast Unit, as he had heard wonderful remarks about them, from his patients.

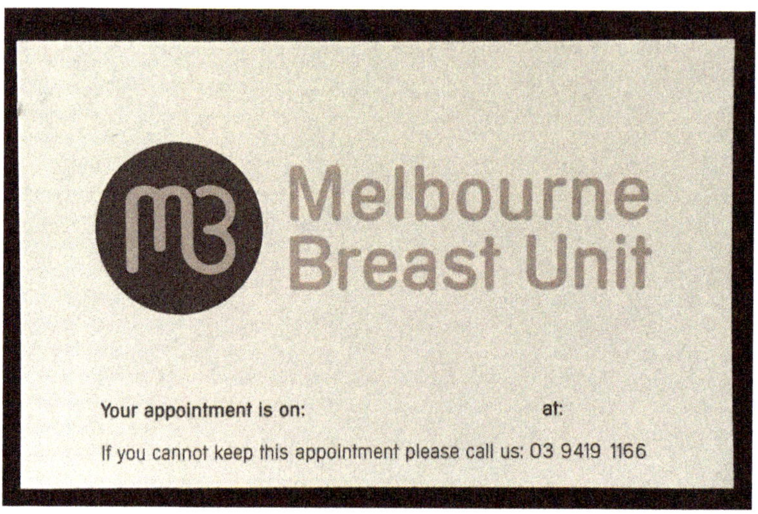

MBU - Melbourne Breast Unit

After explaining my desperate situation to the practice manager of The Melbourne Breast Unit, she insisted that I come to the centre immediately for a consultation with the leading surgeon.

I could not believe my luck and my tears flowed freely. Grateful tears. I have always gone out of my way to help my patients, now, to be on the receiving end, I was truly touched and humbled by the whole experience.

I was fortunate to have the pleasure of meeting Miss Suzanne Neil, the Head Breast Surgeon at The Melbourne Breast Unit.

I had previously heard a lot of positive feedback from patients about Miss Neil and her team. After a thorough examination, she suggested a breast biopsy straight away.

Although she believed that this was, most likely, a benign lump caused by the hormones I was taking, she was aware of the time-critical nature of my problem and decided to obtain a biopsy immediately for a definitive diagnosis.

The whole procedure was over after twenty minutes. I must give credit to the radiologist who performed the biopsy, because the whole procedure, including the local anaesthetic, was virtually painless. After the nurse patched up the wound with some steri-strips, I was ready to go. The result would be available in the afternoon of the very next day. This time, for the first time in years, I hoped and prayed for a negative result.

"Sarah, this is Miss Neil calling. I want to inform you that the biopsy has come out all clear. It is just a proliferation of normal breast tissue, most likely due to the hormones you have been receiving as part of the IVF treatment." Miss Neil had kindly taken the time to call me personally.

I thanked her, and the Melbourne Breast Unit, for their tremendous dedication in supporting women, like myself, during their time of greatest fear. This was truly an amazing Specialist Centre with excellent nursing and radiological support.

Naturally, this roadblock and detour raised the bar of stress and anxiety to another level. I could not believe how unlucky we had been with the cycles. I stopped to give due credit to my family, especially my husband, for his ongoing support and doing whatever he could, in the often difficult task of keeping me sane. I felt truly blessed that we had survived this journey so far. I really hoped that there would soon be a light at the end of this tunnel – a time of joy to reward us all.

Chapter 15: Cycle Number Five, Transfer Number 15

From: Sarah

Subject: Miracle please

Date: 30 June 2013 11:35:29 PM AEST

To: God and baby Babe

Dear God and baby Babe,

The blood test is scheduled for tomorrow and, so far, all the home urine tests have been negative.

I am praying and begging.

Please, please, please...

Love, Sarah

The statistics tell our story and plot our journey to you, Little One...

Failed complete cycles: three

Harvesting procedures: five

Harvested eggs: too many to count

Transfer procedures: seven

Transferred embryos: eight

Our fourth and fifth cycles were known as the back-to-back cycles, so that as many embryos as possible could be collected, biopised and sent to a specialist laboratory in USA. This had to be done within the crucial time frame of eight weeks. Outside that time, the cells would begin to disintegrate.

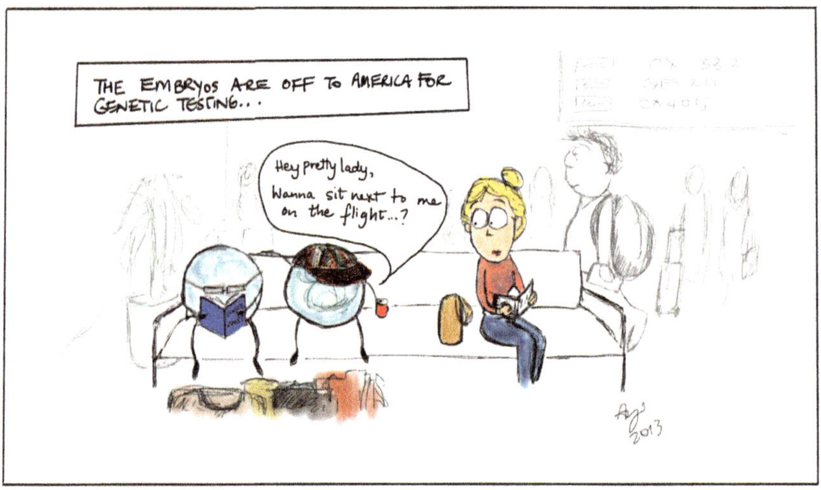
THE EMBRYOS ARE OFF TO AMERICA FOR GENETIC TESTING...
Hey pretty lady, Wanna sit next to me on the flight...?

My sister's cartoon drawing. It cheered me up.

This meant that there were going to be two egg harvests, one immediately after the other. Yes, no rest.

Yes, this also meant a world of medication, side effects, needles, scans, prodding and poking.

The back-to-back cycles were carried out at Clayton campus of Monash IVF. I was introduced to my new IVF nurse, Corrine. She was delightful to work with and she explained everything further in details.

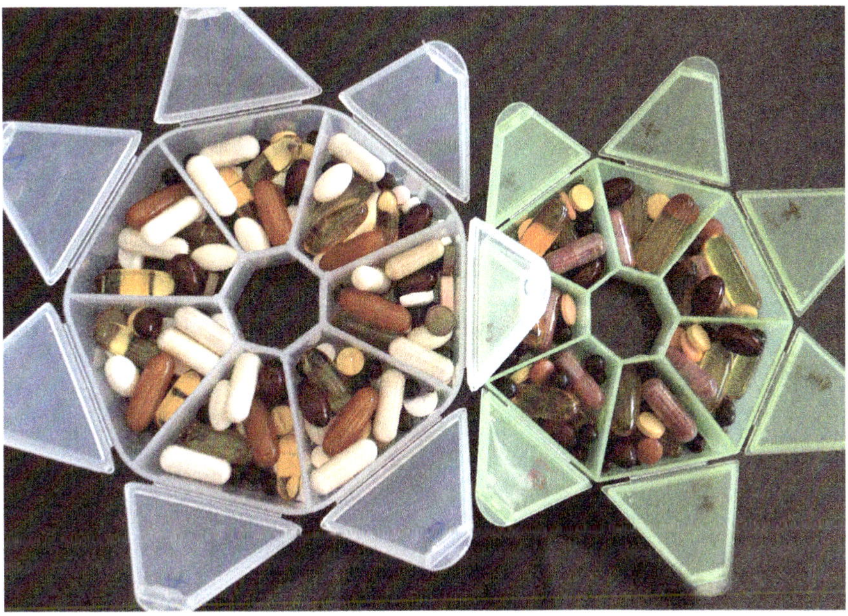

Multi-day Pill boxes. The white box for the morning and the green one for night time. Do you recognise any of these pills?

The first cycle harvest took place on 18 August 2013 and produced five viable day-5 embryos. The following harvest was on 6 October and produced only two. Just one, seemingly like all the others, was transferred on 22 February 2014.

I took a high dose prednisolone as well as Clexane and vaginal progesterone two days before the transfer. I had acupuncture in preparation for, and again after, the transfer.

Then, the usual wait. This time felt different, but perhaps I was kidding myself. Still I had none of the bleeding that has characterised every waiting period to this point. I felt different, but refused to allow myself the hope that had been dashed so many times in the past few years. I waited until the first day that a urinary test would be effective.

Unfortunately, during that time, I caught the flu from your father. Being on steroids had further reduced my immunity; I was feverish with body aches, along with stomach pain and nausea. I convinced myself that every time I coughed, the transferred embryo was one step closer to the exit. I found myself squeezing onto any pelvic floor muscles I could find, just in case this embryo was about to do a runner.

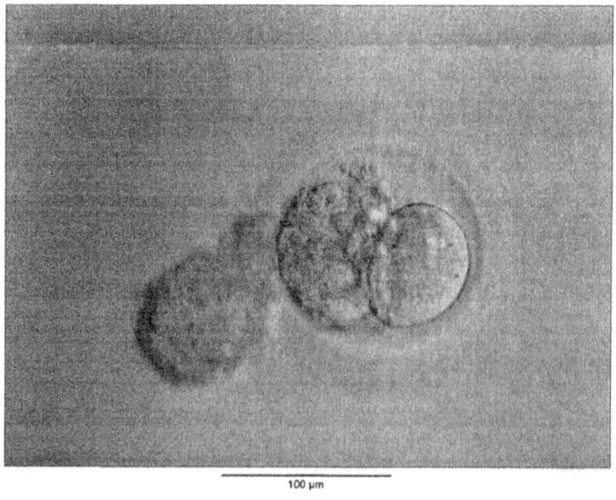

The Day 5 Embryo that was used for the transfer after our back-to-back cycle. The embryologist explained that it was the best one and has already started hatching from its cell.

Sam and I had planned a short trip to Sydney for a conference. Depending on the pregnancy blood test result, it was either going to be a celebratory weekend trip or a few days of silent suffering.

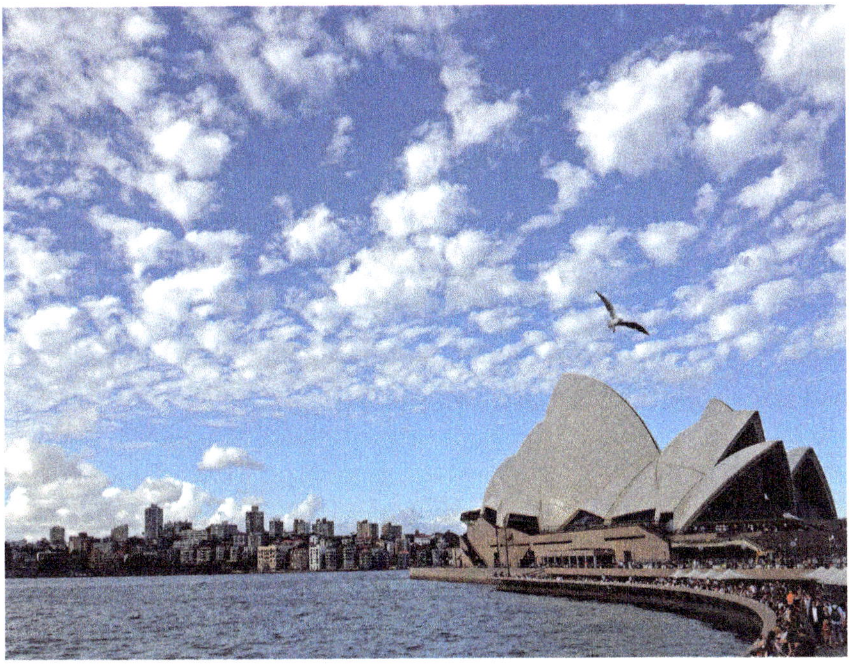

I waited for a long time to take this shot with the seagull soaring just above the Opera House.

The day before the trip, I was scheduled for the pregnancy blood test. As usual, I planned to do a home pregnancy pee test in the morning, prior to seeing the blood nurse.

I have never looked forward to receiving that phone-call from the nurse. Given my track record, I felt it wise to prepare myself.

At six o'clock in the morning, I dragged my body out of the comfort of my cocoon.

Looking at my pale reflection in the mirror, I slipped the plastic strip from the box, as I had done so many times before. As a tsunami of fluid crossed the pregnancy kit viewing-window, my heart pounded and I felt desperately apprehensive – still this was nothing new.

Apprehension and desperation were my default settings at these times. The two-minute wait stretched into what felt like an hour. I could hardly bear to look at the strip and feel that searing pain in my heart again.

One line. Negative, again. I sighed sadly and began to throw the stick into the bin, but I caught sight of something from the corner of my eye. There it was: a very faint red line, parallel to the first, and lazily appearing out of nowhere.

I stopped dead.

I must be imagining it. Could this really be true?

I burst into tears whilst still sitting on the loo. Crying and sobbing like million times before, only these tears were so different. Who knew that a little piece of plastic could create such an outpouring of emotions?

All those years of blood, sweat and tears. All those broken promises and failures. All the sleepless nights and labile emotions.

Finally.

I raided my cupboard in search of other home pregnancy tests.

It took about half a dozen to convince myself. It was unbelievable. We had finally hit the Jackpot!

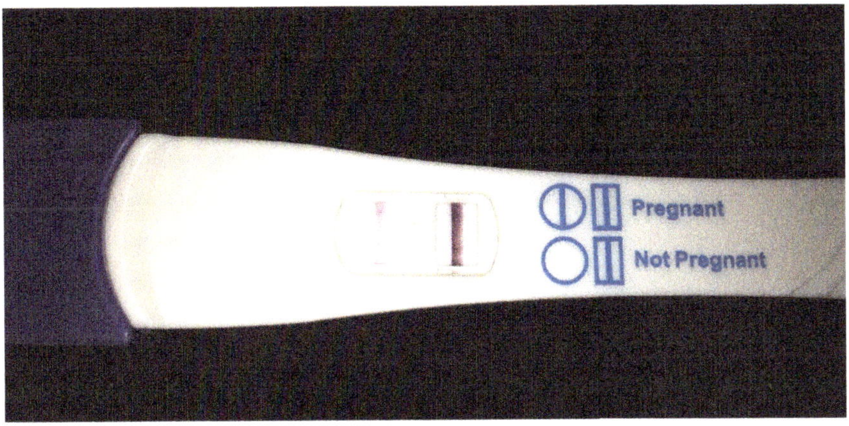

This little stick symbolized many years of blood, sweat and tears.

"What's wrong? Is everything ok? Why are you calling me so early?" Sam was worried as I called on his way to work.

"Honey. I. Am. Pregnant!"

Trying in vain to hold back tears, I broke down over the phone.

There was a momentary silence. We were speechless. A thousand memories from the last seven years flashed before us. We could banish them. Our future would be different.

No more needles. No more invasive tests and surgeries. No more heartache. No more sitting in the waiting rooms. No more crying alone in the shower. No more sobbing in the middle of the night. No more failures. Patience and persistence had ultimately paid off. We could finally walk the red carpet and make our acceptance speech.

The following day, I made the trip to the clinic for the blood test, this time – for the first time – knowing that I had more than hope behind me; this time I had that second, red line to support me, giving me the courage to hope.

The blood taken, I went back to work and tried not to think about the phone call that would tell me the result – that would come later in the day. But when it came, it confirmed everything; Sam and I were having a baby.

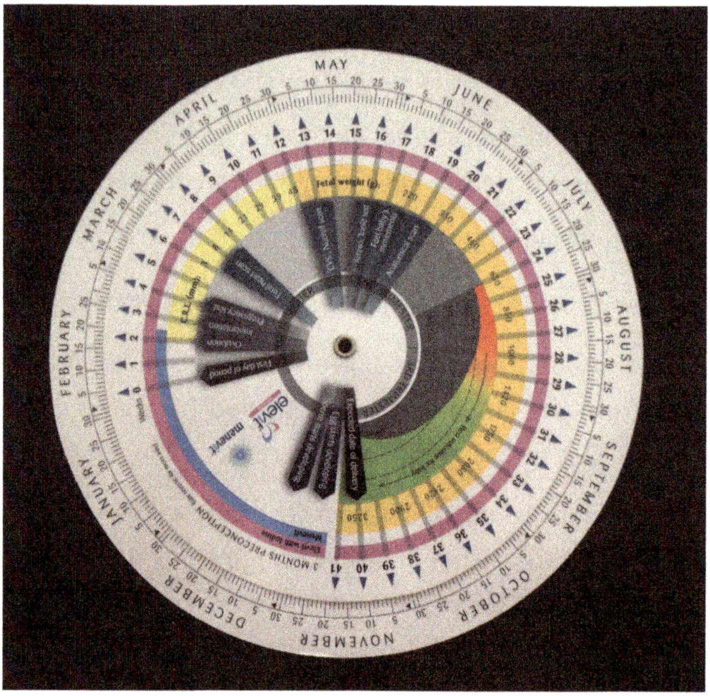

Finally! My own pregnancy wheel. Estimated due date: 11.11.14

Chapter 16: Potential Heartbreak

From: Sarah

Subject: Life can be unfair

Date: 8th April 2014 08:14:11 PM AEST

To: baby Babe

Dear baby Babe,

This is the first time I am writing to you, knowing that you exist inside me.

It is a breathtaking feeling, yet, I am anxious.

You must now realize that your mum is a worrywart. I am nervous about what the future holds and whether we will be perfect parents for you.

We have come a long way and now, we are facing another hurdle. With time, everything will sort itself out.

Don't worry! I promise I will be here for you.

Love, Mummy Sarah

It had finally happened for us – the three of us. You, your dad and I were going to be a family. There is no point in trying to describe how ecstatic we were to know that we only months away from meeting you and being your mum and dad.

The first few weeks were filled with shopping and plans and whole days when we couldn't stop smiling. Our families and friends were so happy for us and the dark years of loss seemed like another planet – one we would never again inhabit.

Those happy weeks numbered exactly seven. I was referred to have the genetic testing by my fertility specialist at the seven-week's check-up.

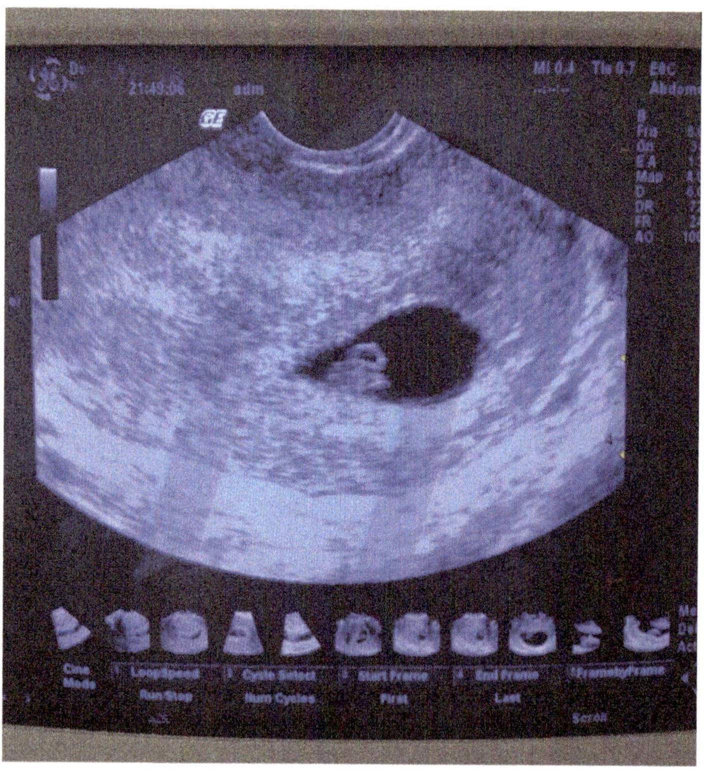

7-weeks Scan at Dr Lynn's Rooms.

I was surprised that this had not been done earlier in, or even prior to, the IVF treatments. When the result came back my world collapsed. I am apparently a carrier for SMA (Spinal Muscular Atrophy). SMA is a terrible condition and affects 1 in 27 Asians. It is a condition of the nervous and muscular system and can be devastating.

There is a spectrum describing the seriousness of how the child will be affected, from mild to severe. Mild cases will be diagnosed in their 30s but will suffer associated significant morbidity with loss of generalised muscle tone. Such people may need walking aids and won't be able to have children. At the severe end of the spectrum, the condition is not compatible with life and these babies often die in utero, or shortly after birth. How could I bear losing you to such a ruinous, shattering diagnosis?

Even though the embryo was biopsied and tested overseas, they were not able to do such a detailed scan, unless we knew specifically which chromosome to target. If we had had this information earlier on, they could have done a more thorough test on chromosome 5, on which the SMA gene defect occurs.

My hopes lay with your father not being a carrier, which would mean that you would have a 50 per cent chance of being a carrier and an equal chance of being unaffected – a healthy little baby. If he was a carrier, there would be a 25 per cent chance of you being affected with SMA, 25 per cent chance normal and 50 per cent still being a carrier. The results of the tests would take a week.

I could not function, that week of the tests, as different outcomes played out my mind. In the worst, blackest moments, I thought of having to have an abortion if the embryo were affected.

I could not imagine myself surviving a termination. Not after all that we had gone through. I swear I lost a few years of my life, dwelling on that blood test result.

Thankfully, it was the good news we had hoped for. Your father had tested negative and was not a carrier.

There were other hurdles, though not quite as terrifying as the possibility of SMA. I had Braxton Hicks contractions quite early in my pregnancy, during second trimester, and again at 36 weeks. These are not of concern once they have been confirmed, but the contractions of early labour had to be ruled out.

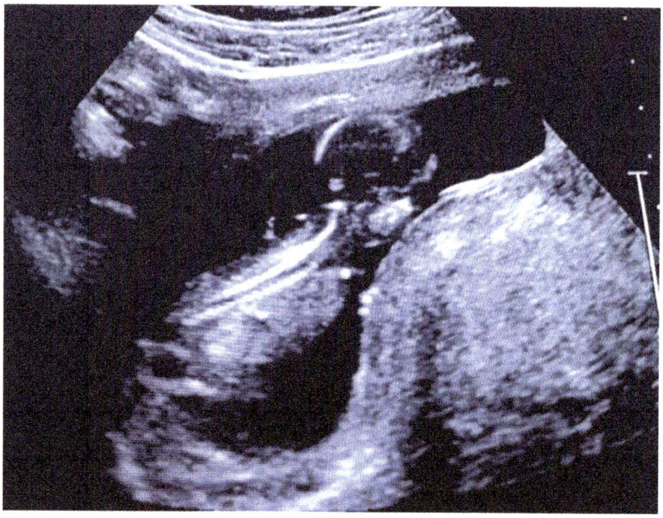

20-weeks Scan at WUME.

Each time I experienced them, I went to hospital for a day's monitoring, and the contractions would settle down. Was it a coincidence that they settled down when I was forced to rest for the monitoring? I think probably not.

I had been working hard and not resting enough when I had the chance.

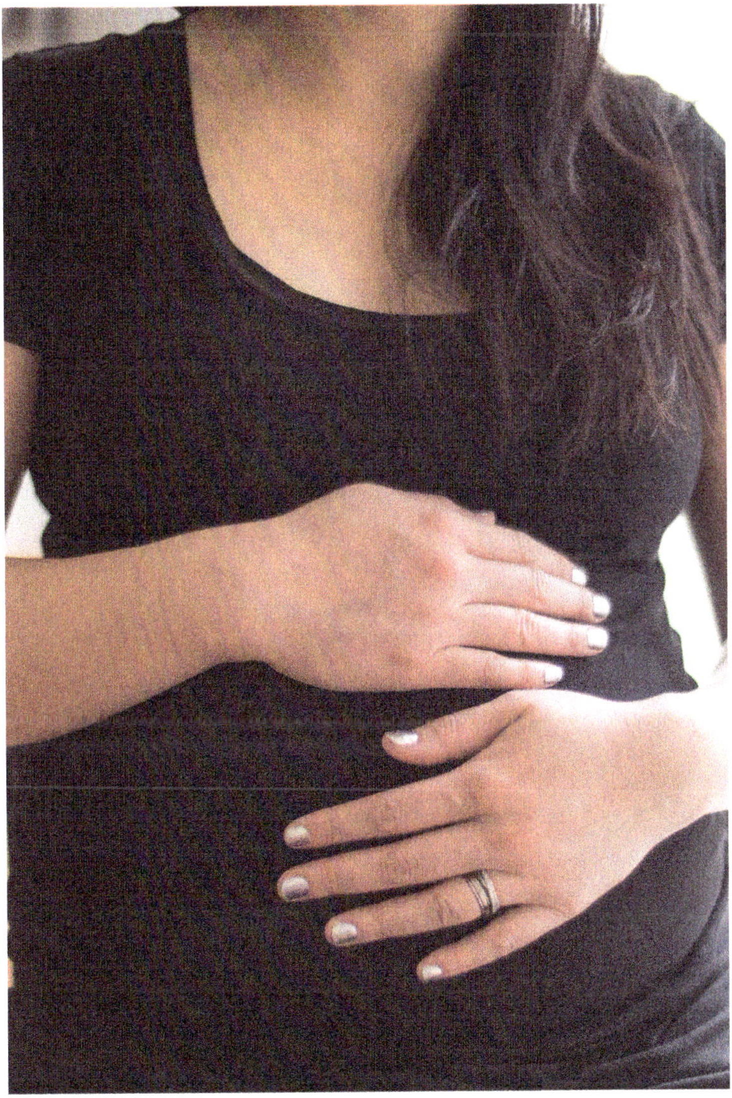

Pregnancy photos by Little Polly Pictures.

With all that had gone before – all the heartache, the tears, and the years of longing – we decided not to chance a normal delivery and planned a caesarean.

This is because, when I was working in the labour ward, a patient delivered a stillborn baby after going through many cycles of IVF. Furthermore, one of my friends had unfortunately suffered the same outcome, when something went wrong with the labour and her little one could not be resuscitated.

These two events had scared me and I didn't want to push my luck. I understood the potential surgical complications, and a longer recovery time, but I held to my decision.

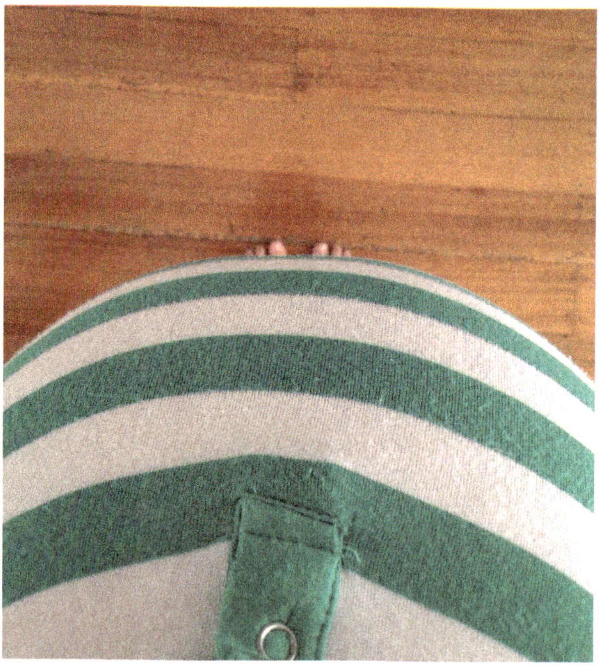

Almost there. Where are my toes?

Chapter 17: Dear Baby Zoe

Dear baby Zoe,

You were born on 6 November 2014.

By now you will know that, but did you know that I wasn't able to hold you within the first few minutes of welcoming you into this World? As soon as the doctor delivered you from my tummy, a bit of air became trapped underneath my breathing muscle, the diaphragm, I have never had such intense chest pain and shoulder tip pain in my life. I thought I was having a heart attack right there on the theatre table.

A quick word from the anaesthetist, not your father, as he was too busy holding and admiring your newborn face, reassured us that I was fine. Being medical, I could only think of the worst but a sneak peek at the anaesthetic monitor revealed a perfect electrocardiograph.

As they placed you on my chest, I sighed with relief and love but took shallow painful breaths whilst posing for the camera. Your voice was loud yet poignant, proving your own existence and announcing your own arrival. While I was being stitched up, your father held you close to my face. I touched your forehead and traced your eyebrows, then down onto your tiny little nose and your petite lips. I couldn't figure out whom you looked like, but I spotted quite quickly that you have my toes and my ears. You were perfect.

Your father stayed so that was our first night as a family.

He did a fantastic job looking after a drowsy new mum in pain and a milk-drunk newborn. I remembered feeling so guilty, when I reluctantly handed you over to the nurse so that your father and I could get some rest that first night. It was at three o'clock in the morning when your bassinet burst into our room, wheeled by one of the nurses. You cried inconsolably. I found you flushed and irritable. You were lying in a pool of sweat and drenched from the humid nursery room. The beanie that I had placed on your little head just a few hours before, to keep you warm, was the main culprit causing you to overheat. Mummy was sorry. I promised you that very night as I whispered into your ears, "Mummy will never leave you in harm's way." I kissed and nursed you, and you took to your feeding immediately. You were a natural. Together, we were adjusting to our new worlds, each with our own set of challenges, you as a newborn and I, as a new mum.

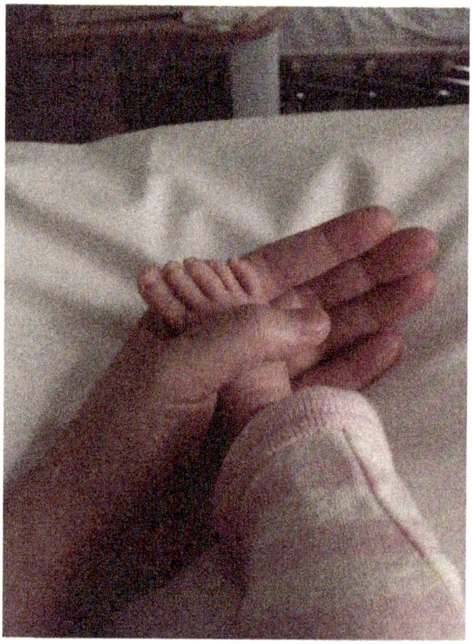

Our first night together in the hospital.

My stay in the hospital was quite a blur. I blamed the painkillers and the noisy environment. I could not get a proper night's rest as I lay awake, unable to sleep because of the other crying babies and sudden bursts of ambulance sirens going back and forth to the hospital. Post-natal blues hit me by surprise on day three after you arrived. It took me a while to recognize what it was, as I was confused as to why I was crying so much. Although the nurses were concerned by my frequent tears, high blood pressure and insomnia, I casually reassured them that everything was fine, because you were sleeping soundly and peacefully by my side. However I did not feel fine. There were times in those first couple of days when I couldn't reach over and comfort you because I was hooked up to the noisy machines. There were times after that when I couldn't reach inside and comfort myself.

The sleep deprivation was slowly destroying my mind and soul. I remember that there was one stretch when I did not sleep for thirty-six hours straight. I was anxious, fatigued and disorientated. When your father had to return to work, I was not coping with looking after you and myself at the same time. I finally succumbed and recognized that I needed help. Luckily your grandparents lived just ten minutes away, so this is where we went to stay, until things improved. We spent your first summer living in your grandparent's home. This was the best decision we could have made. Your father would come over for dinner and play with you before your bedtime. I sobbed when he left for home each night.

Nothing had prepared me for motherhood – certainly not six years of medical school. For the first three months, I grieved for the loss of my independence, my confidence and my pride. I have never felt so lost and guilty.

I was embarrassed that I was not coping – that I was letting everyone down. Friends and family wanted to visit but I politely declined and delayed meeting everyone. I was not physically strong enough to even get out of the house. How could I even think about attending a mother's group and joining other new mums for coffee? Coffee would only make the insomnia worst.

As I lay awake, feeding you, at two and sometimes four o'clock in the morning, I turned to the social media outlet of Facebook. I browsed through photos of new mums enjoying outings with their little ones.

How do they do it? I must be some sort of failure. Some friends left words of encouragement; they said that it would get better. But when?

You teased us with a little smile when you were seven weeks old.

By the end of the three months, you recognized my face and would smile at me whenever I spoke or when I smiled down at you. I felt our unique connection and bond.

Suddenly, the self-doubting insecurity fog lifted and I started to feel better. I could read your baby body language better, and my intuition would guide me along the way. For the first time, I felt confident that I could be the mother you needed and that we would both enjoy our special bond immensely.

Zoe. How I love calling your name, Zoe. I am still pinching myself at the realisation that you are finally here. You missed the Stork Express a couple of times but not to worry, we waited patiently for you and we were rewarded by you, our perfect little daughter.

Do you know how we chose your name?

Because we knew you were going to be a girl, we were able to narrow it down to four names a few weeks before you were born. Rebecca, Chloe, Jasmine and Zoe. Each morning, we read the names aloud and we decided to name you Zoe. I had already picked the Chinese middle names for you. Don't you worry. Mummy will teach you how to write your name in both English and Chinese when you are a little bit older.

But there is a more significant reason we chose it – another story to your name. One of my clients, who shares the same birth name as you, has helped me tremendously with prayers. She also guided me with spiritual support throughout the years whilst we were undergoing fertility treatments. Around that time, she travelled to Malta for a pilgrimage and visited her cousin, who was the head of a convent. She prayed to Blessed Adeodata Pisani for us, and introduced me to her story and veneration. I must admit I wasn't as religious I used to be.

Given what we had gone through, we had lost a lot of faith. I saw it as a punishment for something that I must have done in the past.

After that terrible incident at Christmas in 2012, I had even stopped asking for miracle. This loyal customer approached me one day and asked if I was open to her praying for us. I could sense the hesitancy in her voice. Something inside me changed when I accepted her offer. I was touched by her sincerity and, over time, she has rekindled my broken spirit. I believed in her. I considered her The Messenger. I didn't tell this story to your father until the day when we finally decided that her name would be your name, Zoe. Coincidence or not, I believed there was a Higher Power watching over and looking after us.

Let me teach you something, Zoe. To keep someone in your prayers over a period of time is a very noble and selfless act. To accept prayers on your behalf, you ought to learn to be humble and acknowledge the fact that you need help. There are times where denial and anger has taken the better of me. As your mother, I am not perfect, but through these obstacles, resilience found me. At the end of the day, you have to keep searching for inner peace and love. I am very lucky, because I found both when I cradled you in my arms.

Perhaps you are too young to understand how much we love you. There aren't enough fingers and toes to count. No calculator can arrive at a large enough figure. I hope that, one day, you will also be able to experience this unique bond with your own child. Despite losing track of time, second-guessing myself, losing my identity and sanity, there is this unimaginable pleasure that comes from fulfilment and serenity.

As I emerge as a new mum, guided by the sleepless nights and your never-ending feeds, I can only describe what I do and how I feel. This is maternal love: it is a constant longing. It is an unspoken connection that is bonded by blood, sweat, tears, joy and time. It is an overwhelming feeling of vulnerability that consumes my every breathing moment. It is in the endless tasks of changing, feeding and burping into the darkest hour of the night.

It's when I forget all the pain of the journey and, in the wee hours of the morning, I find myself singing, hushing, and dancing to an unheard melody with you in my aching arms.

Dear Zoe, this is unconditional love.

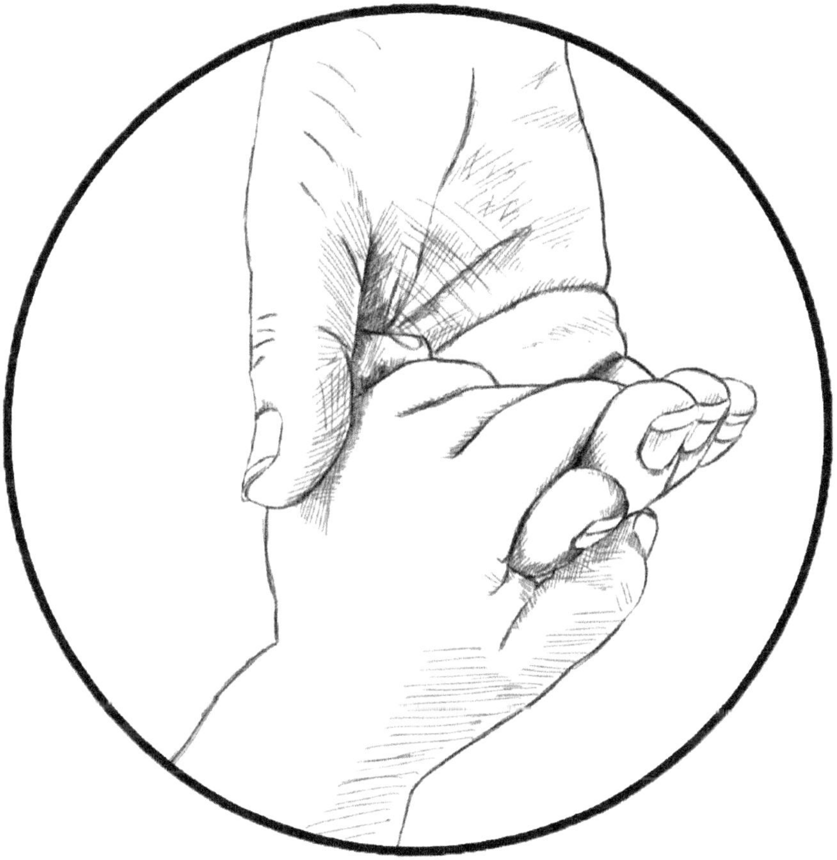

Illustrated by Little Polly Pictures

About the Author

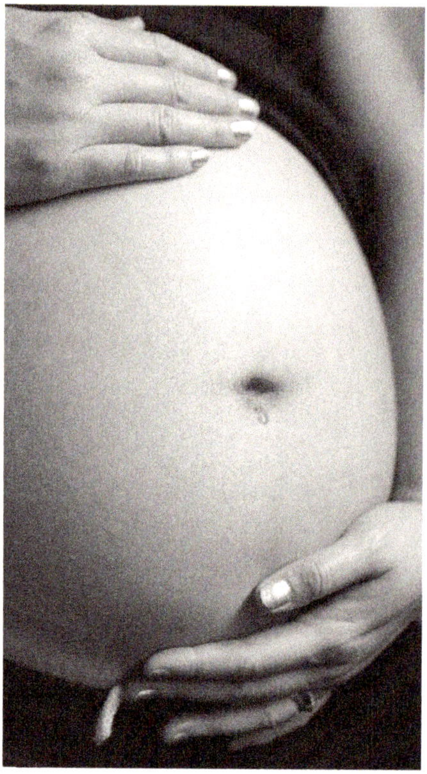

Pregnancy photos by Little Polly Pictures.

Dr Sarah Lnyy is a qualified General Practitioner, Living in Melbourne, Australia and holds a Diploma in Obstetrics with the Royal Australia and New Zealand College of Obstetricians and Gynaecologists. Her special interests include skin cancer and aesthetic medicine, student health, women's health, pregnancy-care and massage therapy in general practice. As a writer, she has several articles published in various medical journals.

In 2011, Sarah and her husband began their IVF journey. The stress and solitude of having these treatments led the author to change her career path. She resigned from General Practice in late 2012 and acquired a small business in beauty therapy and aesthetic medicine.

Dr Sarah Lnyy is passionate about learning and teaching. She has recently completed the Certificate IV in Training and Assessment, with the goal of providing quality training to staff members in the medical aesthetic field.

As a medical doctor, she encountered many heart-breaking life and death situations. As an aesthetic doctor, she sees the wisdom and beauty in every face. As an IVF patient, she has first-hand experience and insight into the emotional roller coaster of seeking fertility treatments.

In her spare time, she enjoys spending time with her family, sewing, knitting, baking and cooking with the Thermomix.

Sarah and Sam are pleased to announce that Zoe will be expecting a sibling in late November 2016.

Connect with Sarah

www.drsarahlnyy.com.au

https://www.facebook.com/DrSarahLnyy

sarahlnyy@gmail.com

Other Books from Dreamstone Publishing

Dreamstone publishes books in a wide variety of categories – here are some of our other bestselling books:-

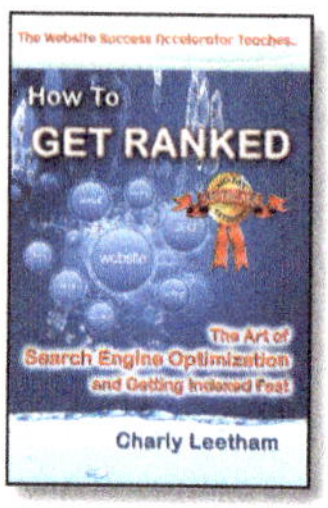

Get Ranked
The Art of Search Engine Optimisation and Getting Indexed Fast
(The Website Success Accelerator Teaches...)

By Charly Leetham

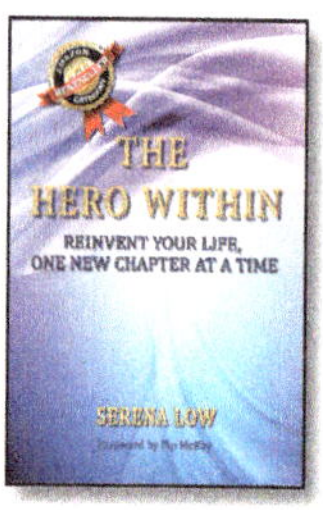

The Hero Within
Reinvent Your Life, One New Chapter at a Time

By Serena Low

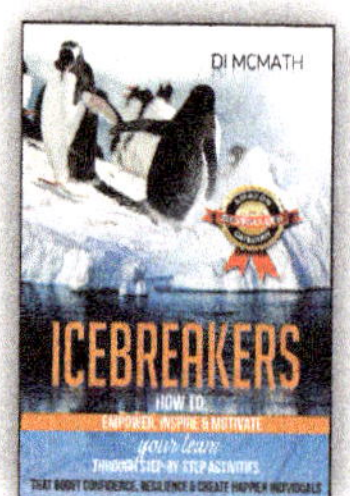

"Icebreakers : How to Empower, Motivate and Inspire Your Team, Through Step-by-Step Activities That Boost Confidence, Resilience and Create Happier Individuals"

By Di McMath

Be first to know when our next books are coming out – sign up for our newsletter at

http://www.dreamstonepublishing.com

CPSIA information can be obtained
at www.ICGtesting.com
Printed in the USA
BVOW10s0032090816
4458BVAU00002B/2/P

9 781925 165944